Default Caregivers

Default Caregivers

Jean Setne

authorHOUSE®

AuthorHouse™
1663 Liberty Drive
Bloomington, IN 47403
www.authorhouse.com
Phone: 1-800-839-8640

Some names and identifying details have been changed to protect the privacy of individuals. This book is not intended as a substitute for the medical advice of physicians. The reader should regularly consult a physician in matters relating to his/her health and particularly with respect to any symptoms that may require diagnosis or medical attention.

First published by AuthorHouse : 06/06/2011

ISBN: 978-1-4567-6699-3 (sc)
ISBN: 978-1-4567-6698-6 (dj)
ISBN: 978-1-4567-6697-9 (ebk)

Library of Congress Control Number: 2011906085

Printed in the United States of America

Any people depicted in stock imagery provided by Thinkstock are models, and such images are being used for illustrative purposes only.

Certain stock imagery © Thinkstock.

This book is printed on acid-free paper.

Because of the dynamic nature of the Internet, any web addresses or links contained in this book may have changed since publication and may no longer be valid. The views expressed in this work are solely those of the author and do not necessarily reflect the views of the publisher, and the publisher hereby disclaims any responsibility for them.

CONTENTS

For Marilyn with love.

And for Paul, without whose encouragement this book would not have been possible.

Disclaimer

Some names and identifying details have been changed to protect the privacy of individuals

Acknowledgements

The author wishes to acknowledge her relatives and friends who read early drafts.

Also, many thanks to the non-fiction writers in the Mesilla Valley Writers group, whose guidance and support was invaluable.

Chapter 1

ER

Karen was sharing her home with her sister Penny, who had arrived just before Christmas. Karen had been diagnosed with Hepatitis C seven years earlier. She had contracted it when she received platelet transfusions nearly twenty years earlier. Her liver function had been monitored since then. A few months before her sister moved in with her, a local gastroenterologist advised Karen her liver disease had worsened. The doctor referred her to Mayo Clinic in Phoenix. At Mayo, Karen had undergone a thorough evaluation and had been registered on a liver transplant waiting list. That was back in September.

But her condition had continued in a downward spiral, and by December she could no longer live alone. Penny came to her sister's aid, moving in to help her through her illness, doing the cooking, cleaning and driving, while they waited for a transplant.

The holidays were over, and it was a Friday, January 20th. Penny noticed her sister, who hadn't had much energy for several weeks, was "acting weird." Karen was slurring her words and acting extremely lethargic. In the late afternoon Penny prepared some soup. The next thing she remembered was Karen's face in her bowl of soup! Penny tried to get her sister up to her feet so they could walk to the car in the garage, a distance of perhaps 30 feet. But Karen was too weak, and fell to the floor.

With the help of a next-door neighbor, Penny finally got her sister into the car. Next she called Norma, a cousin of Karen's husband, Dave, and asked Norma if she would go with her to the nearest Emergency

Room. Penny drove to Norma's house, and the two women took Karen to the ER in Tucson, Arizona, some 32 miles from Karen's home in Green Valley, Arizona. During the car ride, Karen did not know where she was or where they were headed. As they drove, Norma had to keep reminding her where they were going.

At the emergency room Karen was treated for constipation and what we had come to know as a high level of ammonia, which affected her brain. The symptoms of this condition, which I later learned is called hepatic encephalopathy, are confusion, lethargy, brain fog, and muscle weakness, all of which Penny witnessed in her sister that day. It was clear Karen had not been taking her prescription medication as recommended. A person with liver disease needs assistance in controlling toxins that build up, among them ammonia. When a person's liver is badly diseased, a prescription laxative called Lactulose is used to remove ammonia and other toxins from the digestive tract (since the liver is not working). Karen's dosage of the laxative, which she had been taking for a number of years, had recently been increased from once daily at bedtime to three or four doses daily.

That January it is likely Karen had cut her dosage to one per day, as once daily had been her regular dosage when she first started taking it so many years before. Or, quite possibly, because of not being able to *remember* whether she had taken it or not, she might have stopped taking it altogether.

It was several hours at the Emergency Room before Karen knew where she was and "became herself" again. The staff at the ER treated her symptoms and, much later that evening, sent her home.

Penny and Karen's brother Paul is my husband. Paul and I had been in nearly daily contact with his sisters after Penny moved in during December. We heard about the trip to the ER a few days after it happened.

On Friday, January 27, Penny called Paul at our home in Alamogordo, New Mexico. Penny said, "Paul, our sister is pretty bad." She went on to say she had already called Karen's Transplant Nurse Coordinator at Mayo, Jack Kelly, and described the latest symptoms. Jack had told Penny how Karen needed to be treated at the ER. Penny told us she had just watched as Karen was driven away in an ambulance, which she had summoned. Penny said she was preparing to follow in the car in a few minutes.

"This is getting to be a weekly experience," she continued, with panic rising in her voice. She explained about Karen's muscle weakness and brain fog, and assured us she wouldn't be calling unless she thought it was necessary. She finally said, "Come to Tucson and meet me at the Emergency Room, can you, can you come?"

As I began to pack a couple of small bags, I heard Paul soothe his eldest sister over the phone. He said we would be on our way shortly, and in the meantime she needed to try to calm down. He added, "When you think you are ready, you need to drive very carefully." I heard Paul caution her about evening rush-hour traffic. Paul's soothing words were what his sister needed to hear. Over the preceding eight or nine days she had witnessed a significant change in her sister's condition. She was frightened, and wanted us to see firsthand what was happening.

It was after 10:30 p.m. when we met Penny in the parking lot of the hospital. She said Karen was just starting to talk normally. When we asked what exactly had happened, she said they had been sitting in the living room. When Karen tried to stand she could not raise herself out of the chair or trust her legs to hold her once she was standing. Like the week before, Penny was afraid Karen would fall to the floor, and knew she did not have the strength to lift her. Telling her sister to stay put, she decided she had better call an ambulance. Paul assured Penny she had done the right thing; how could she have done anything else?

Then Penny wanted us to know what the attending physician said to her. She said, "There was a doctor in the emergency room that seemed to be unfamiliar with Hepatitis C and liver disease. He scolded me for calling an ambulance. So I explained that elevated ammonia is one of the side effects of a malfunctioning liver and that it causes brain fog and weakness in muscles and joints. I told him Karen couldn't get out of her chair or stand or walk. I explained that it was my understanding that Karen needed to be treated to get her toxin levels down."

Penny continued, "I thought I heard the doctor mumble something to the effect of, 'She's in liver failure and she's going to die.' Those are fighting words!" Penny exclaimed.

With that, Penny became strong and assertive, actually more like a mother lion with her cubs. She said she told the doctor, in no uncertain terms, that her sister was on the national transplant list and awaiting surgery at Mayo in Phoenix.

"She has plans *to live*, not to die," she pointed out. Penny urged the doctor to change his thinking.

"Good for you, Penny!" I thought.

Once in the ER, Paul and I talked to Karen for a short while. She seemed tired but unaware of the drama that had just occurred. Paul suggested to Penny that she should drive back to the house and try to get some rest. Since she was several steps past the point of exhaustion, she agreed. She reminded us she would have to wait up to buzz us into the gated community in Green Valley. A short while later Paul and I were told Karen was going to be admitted to the hospital overnight. Then we also drove to the house. We all finally turned in for some rest at 1:30 a.m.

During that short night of sleep I dreamed about Karen. She was walking toward me with a spring in her step. She was thin and smiling. She was walking next to a long, white building, which I didn't recognize. None of it made sense.

Karen spent the weekend in the hospital. On Monday, January 30th, a doctor in Karen's room talked with Karen, Penny, Paul, and me. He said he was going to have to release Karen and wanted to know what our plans were. We knew she was too weak to be at home; we knew her care was too much for Penny to handle on her own. Paul asked what some alternatives for his sister's care might be.

One suggestion was that she could enter a health care facility where the staff could help her regain her strength and her ability to walk. For the next few hours, a wonderful, resourceful man phoned various facilities in the area and contacted Karen's insurance company to be certain the proposed stay would be covered. To this day I do not know his name or title. He was one of the many unknown and tremendously talented professionals who helped during Karen's illness.

While the gentleman was working on her behalf, Karen had a meltdown. By then she knew she was very sick. After just three days in the hospital, she was even weaker than she had been a few days earlier. She hadn't been up and walking around her hospital room; she was flat on her back in bed. She wailed, "I can't go home. Nobody wants me.

Where will I go?" Penny looked at Paul. Paul looked at Penny and me. I went over to Karen's bed and took her hand in mine.

I looked her in the eye and said, "We will find you a place. This is just temporary. Look at all the things you've been through in your life. This is just a bump in the road. You can do this. You are so strong. It won't be long before you'll be looking back on this and realizing it wasn't so bad." She stared into my eyes, held on tight, and began to nod. I hoped what I was saying would be true. Minutes later we learned the name of the facility that had a room for her.

Chapter 2

Karen's Background

Karen Lea Henley was born in 1942. Karen married Dave King in November 1961 at the age of 19, just a few months after meeting him in an automotive parts store in Phoenix. She went into the store to buy car wax for her Corvette. The two started talking, and she learned Dave also owned a Corvette. Dave offered to help Karen wax her car. They made a date to meet later. When she walked out to the parking lot where her girlfriend was waiting, Karen said, "I just met the guy I'm going to marry."

Karen was a petite woman at 5' 3" tall, and she had a tiny waist. She had dark brown hair, and took great care and a lot of time with her hairstyles. She had dark eyes and wore glasses. She applied makeup carefully "so her eyes wouldn't get lost behind her glasses." She was a feminine woman. People called her glamorous.

Karen's older sister, Penny, had been married two years earlier. Penny had her first child in 1960 and was busy raising her family. Their younger brother, Paul, had just graduated from high school in the spring of 1961. Paul went to college in New York, attending the same college his father had attended. The three teenagers had been extremely close as children, having been born within 28 months when their parents were young. They had played together and had gone to school together; in fact sometimes Penny and Karen had been in the same classroom. The death of their father in 1960 had set them all on their own separate life paths, scattering the members of the family.

Karen's mother Josephine suddenly found herself a widow and a single Mom, raising five-year-old Susan and three-year-old Allen. Karen thought of the two younger ones as "the second family" since there were fourteen years between her and her younger sister, and 16 years between her and her youngest brother. Josephine moved to South Dakota in 1961 with the young children, less than a year after the death of her husband, to finish some work he had started there.

Karen and Dave welcomed their first child, a girl, in October 1962. Lea favored her father in looks, with beautiful strawberry blonde hair. She became a very talkative child, a trait she got from both her parents. Her little brother Randy came along three years later, in October 1965. He looked like Karen's side of the family, with dark brown hair and huge dark brown eyes. Randy was a sickly baby and required a lot of his mother's attention for many years when he was young.

The family spent many years in the Phoenix area. Dave progressed through his sales career in the automotive parts business. His job required him to be away from home a lot during the week, and usually at home on weekends. As a result Karen became very competent, handling the children's scraped knees and other small childhood emergencies on her own.

When the family schedule permitted, Karen did some fashion modeling, sold jewelry and cosmetics, or worked part-time jobs in the evenings. Her primary focus at the time, though, was the children. She kept her home spotless and her children neat, clean and well cared for.

Twenty-three years later.

It was the fall of 1985. Karen was 43 and her children were grown. During the passing years, Dave's career had required the family to move from Phoenix, Arizona to Pennsylvania, and in 1980, from Pennsylvania to the Jackson, Mississippi area. Karen attended college there; finishing the degree she had begun after high school. She enrolled for 19 hours in the fall term, knowing she would complete all requirements for graduation just before Christmas.

Karen was both challenged and excited about her heavy class load. Something of a perfectionist, she spent many hours doing homework, writing papers, reading and studying. She didn't let any of her other duties as wife, mother, cook, and homemaker slip, either. Thanksgiving and Christmas arrived, and she decorated her home lavishly for the holidays.

She got very little sleep. During that period, Karen took less time than normal with her appearance, as she often had to dash out the door at the last minute to attend a class. She knew she was run-down, but she also knew the end of the busy college term was in sight.

In December, she noticed the left side of her neck was horribly swollen. She made arrangements to see a doctor, and tests were scheduled. She had exploratory surgery on her abdomen. Her medical team determined she had Hodgkin's disease, and it was in Stage III-B. The diagnosis meant this cancer, also known as Hodgkin's Lymphoma[1] was in her lymph nodes above and below her diaphragm. In short, it was likely the cancer had spread pretty much throughout her body.

Karen had another surgery in January 1986, during which some lymph nodes in her abdomen were removed. Her spleen was also removed. Dave called Penny and asked for her help. Without hesitating, she rushed to her sister's side to nurse her through her recovery. Fortunately, Karen healed quickly from both of these surgeries.

Then chemotherapy treatment began for the cancer remaining in other parts of her body. Since the cancer was so far advanced, and the chemotherapy treatments were harsh, Karen's body would have had a hard time fighting any infections. She was told not to risk having contact with people other than her family and a close circle of friends. She said she felt like she'd been given a sentence of "house arrest." She was warned she would probably lose her hair. Almost immediately, her hair started to come out in clumps. Karen and her next-door neighbor went out for a quick trip to a wig shop.

Karen was angry. She struggled through a period of time when she was thinking "why me?" Her life had been going well, her children were on their own. She had just completed her college classes for a degree and then, boom, cancer. It didn't seem fair and she was not happy. She didn't want to be confined to her home for a long period of time, she didn't want to lose her hair, and she didn't want to be sick.

Shortly after Lea learned her mother had cancer, she decided to locate her mother's brother, Uncle Paul, even though her mother and the other siblings had not been in touch very much during the previous fifteen years or so. The last time Paul had seen Lea she had been a small child. She remembered hearing stories about how her mother,

Aunt Penny and Uncle Paul had been close as little kids. Lea felt her uncle would want to know her mother's condition.

Karen was really pleased with the reunion her daughter arranged. Penny was living in Texas at the time. Paul had moved many times since he left Arizona. Lea remembered knowing he'd been in Minneapolis years before. Using directory assistance and the help of a telephone operator, as this was years before the Internet or tools like Google were available, Lea obtained Paul's phone number. She realized good luck was on her side; Minneapolis was the first city she called, thinking perhaps he had been there all along. It was also news to her and the rest of the family that Paul was engaged to me.

So, at Lea's urging and as a gift to Karen in May 1986, Penny, Paul and I gathered in Mississippi for Karen's graduation from college. Susan, their younger sister, and a cousin, Julie, also arrived for the weekend. Karen was receiving chemotherapy treatments, but she was doing pretty well. She had been given permission to attend her college commencement ceremony, and to have a small gathering at her home that evening. She surprised us all when she appeared in her back yard wearing a pink synthetic wig. It was her way of saying cancer wasn't going to rob her of her sense of humor! She said, "If having cancer is what it took to get us all back together, then it was worth it."

Shortly after the visit from so many family members, Karen arrived at a feeling of acceptance about the cancer. She became determined to fight it. Paul discussed the power of the mind-body connection, as well as some visualization techniques, to marshal her energy at all times to battle the cancer cells.

Chapter 3

Back in Tucson, Present Time

Twenty years after her fight with Hodgkin's disease, Karen again needed to summon her energy and focus on fighting for her life. We accompanied her as she checked into a rehabilitation center in Tucson, Arizona on Monday, January 30, 2006. Acting as her spokesperson, Penny described Karen's condition as she had observed it over the previous couple of weeks. Paul, too, indicated to the staff that our main concern was that Karen had to become able to walk again following the decline that had so quickly followed the episodes that landed her in the emergency room.

The people in the physical therapy department at the nursing home went to work. Karen was started on the road to getting her strength back; she needed to overcome the muscle weakness that came with such high levels of toxins. Once again Penny contacted Jack Kelly, Karen's transplant nurse coordinator at Mayo in Phoenix, so he would know Karen's condition and where she was residing for the time being.

Paul drove home to New Mexico the next day. He and I had decided I would stay with Penny in Arizona for a few days so the two of us could look in on Karen together. Penny needed the companionship. Even though Paul and I had kept in touch regularly with his sisters by phone, Penny felt like she had been single-handedly carrying the care load on her shoulders for more than six weeks. So Penny and I visited Karen together each day, and I did all the driving that week. I was able to cook a few simple meals, and do some of the laundry. Penny was able to put her feet up and relax a bit, both mentally and physically, while we shared the space in Karen's house.

After hearing from Penny, Jack Kelly had been in contact with the staff at the nursing home there in Tucson, instructing them on the needs of a patient with advanced liver disease. On February 1, 2006 Penny and I learned Karen was receiving four doses, as prescribed, of the laxative medication daily. Karen wasn't happy about the related numerous trips to the bathroom. But we were all reassured that she was getting the proper amount of medication and we hoped the confusion, lethargy, and muscle weakness associated with the hepatic encephalopathy were a thing of the past.

By Saturday, February 4 Karen was proudly reporting on her physical therapy progress. She was walking with a walker and gaining strength in her legs, as well as some confidence in her *ability* to walk. Paul drove back from New Mexico to Arizona that day to pick me up. He and I realized Karen was in good hands, and that Penny's stress level had come down somewhat since Karen had moved into the nursing home. We told Karen not to expect Penny to visit every day while at the same time encouraged Penny to give herself a day off as often as she needed from the 70-mile round-trip drive to Tucson. Both sisters, it seemed, were in a better place after the frightening recent trips to the emergency room. It was shocking to realize Karen would not have made it if Penny had not been with her to transport her to the ER the first week and to summon the ambulance to transport her the second week.

We kept in contact with Penny by phone. By February 10, there was talk that Karen was going to be released the following week. A lot of progress had been made in just a dozen days. Everyone was encouraged by what seemed to be a positive new phase.

However, on February 12 a blood clot was discovered behind the knee in Karen's left leg. The doctor ordered Karen to begin complete bed rest; even bathroom privileges were not allowed. I never heard anyone talk about the risk of the blood clot moving to Karen's lungs, but that possibility was on our minds. A week later the staff arranged for Karen to be transported to the hospital, where a Greenfield filter was inserted in Karen's portal vein, which carries blood from the legs back to the heart. The filter's job was to prevent any blood clots from the legs from moving up to the heart or lungs. When Karen was released to go back to the nursing home, she was again ordered to complete bed rest for an indefinite amount of time. The walking strength she had gained was slipping away. Someone told me for every day a person stays in bed, it takes two days to recover. In Karen's case, I feared it might be a one-day-to-three or one-day-to-four ratio to come back.

Penny continued her regular treks to Tucson to see her sister. During the same period, that is, the first couple of weeks of February, Jack Kelly advised Penny, Paul, and me that Karen's children should be summoned to come and visit their mother. This was a jolt as we began to realize what Jack was telling us. His years of experience with other liver transplant candidates indicated these setbacks were extremely serious. He no doubt had first-hand knowledge of how much or how often a patient is able (or ultimately not able) to recover from them.

Penny and Paul began to make regular contact with Karen's children, then ages 43 and 40. They had the delicate job of asking Lea and Randy to come, while not wanting to alarm them too much about the various issues, such as Karen's brain fog and confusion, her lack of mobility, and the blood clot, to name a few. Paul told Lea there were so many potentially life-threatening issues that both she and Randy should make plans to come to Arizona.

It seemed to me Lea and Randy had a difficult time understanding the serious nature of their mother's condition. The last time they had seen their Mom she was "about the same," "hanging in there" with her liver disease, something she had been dealing with for more than six years. They had been keeping in touch with their mother by phone. Whenever they asked, Karen would say she was "pretty good." Karen had adopted a practice of not complaining much, and likely had not told her children that she had gotten worse. So it must have seemed sudden and incomprehensible that their Mom was in a nursing home, on forced bed-rest, unable to walk. Both of Karen's children lived in other states, and had various reasons why it would have been difficult to come to Arizona for a visit. Even when Paul suggested that they might have to suffer the consequences of their choices if he had to call and announce the time for her funeral, Lea kept saying, "I know my mother; she's going to be alright." Lea seemed confident (or possibly was in denial). Penny, Paul, and I no longer had that certainty; we had seen Karen's condition deteriorate and we had heard Jack's repeated warnings.

Chapter 4

Medical History and How Karen Got Hepatitis

I met Karen and her family for the first time during her college graduation weekend in May 1986. She impressed me with her sense of humor and strength as she faced her cancer challenge. She talked constantly. She was easy to be with and seemed happiest when engaging someone in conversation. Dave was the funniest person I had ever met, finding humor in everything. He could tell jokes and stories for every occasion, and entertained us all.

Penny told me years later that she and Karen liked me instantly. They agreed that weekend to "adopt me" as another sister. On Sunday as Paul and I prepared to return to Minneapolis, we promised to stay in touch with Karen, Dave, Lea and Randy, as well as Penny and the rest of the family members. Paul and I were married in August that year. Due to her on-going chemotherapy treatments, Karen and her family were unable to attend our wedding.

A few days after a routine blood draw and lab tests in June 1986, Karen received a phone call.

"Come to the hospital right away," she was told. "Don't take time to pack a bag, change your clothes, or take a shower. Come immediately, and have your husband drive you here."

Being a habitual night owl and late riser, Karen was likely still dressed in a nightgown and robe. It didn't matter. She and Dave rushed to the hospital as instructed. She learned that her white blood count had dropped to zero. It was a count that would have to be up at 1,000 in order to get her next chemotherapy treatment. Chemotherapy lowers levels of healthy blood cells, but this was dangerous! She was put into isolation. The slightest infection or illness could have killed her.

She received a transfusion of platelets. Platelets are the blood components that cause the blood to clot. Like the white blood count, the platelets were dangerously low. After one transfusion Karen had a severe reaction, with chills and shaking uncontrollably. She could not get warm, even with several blankets. Slowly the white blood count and platelet count rose, and she came out of it.

Blood was not screened for hepatitis in the spring of 1986. Routine testing of the US blood supply began in 1990[2], although testing was only for Hepatitis B. While still in the hospital, Karen was informed she had contracted hepatitis from the platelets transfusions she had received. Less was known about hepatitis at that time. She was understandably not at her best when she was given this information. She was being treated for cancer and had gone through a dangerous period of low blood counts because of that treatment, not to mention her reaction to the transfusions. She heard plainly that she had hepatitis, that she would need to tell her regular doctors that she did, and that she shouldn't take aspirin ever again.

Karen was a good patient, and listened to the instructions carefully. At that time, no one spoke about future implications associated with the new information regarding hepatitis.

Besides, Karen had Hodgkin's disease then. She was focused on what she needed to do to get better, that was her immediate concern.

Karen's blood count finally rose to 1,000. At the end of June 1986 she was released from the hospital. The platelets she had been given saved her from the brink of the frightening "zero blood count" episode.

Her battle against cancer waged on.

In fact, it was another five months before Karen received her final chemotherapy treatment. Through all that time, she focused her energy on getting her health back. Indeed, after fighting Hodgkin's for nearly a year, she was told at the end of 1986 she was cancer-free.

She was proud of herself and she had good reason to be. She had stayed the course through many hospitalizations and extremely difficult chemotherapy treatments. She had taught herself, her children and others that cancer was not always a death sentence. She was well.

Life for Karen returned to normal. She had earned a Bachelor of Science degree with a major in Business Administration and a concentration in Finance. She was ready and eager to leave her house and get out into the world again. Her hair grew back and for the first time in her life, it was curly! She was slim and attractive. She again enjoyed her great sense of fashion and style. She knew how to add an extra bit of pizzazz to an outfit with a scarf, an interesting piece of jewelry, or a pair of earrings that enhanced her coloring. She usually had long, carefully shaped fingernails, which she kept polished.

The year was 1987 and Karen went to work in an insurance agency. She obtained her securities license as well as licenses in life and health insurance and in annuities. In 1989 she became the first Planning Specialist at a financial planning firm. She had found a niche where her expertise from her college courses, her licensure, and her math and computer skills could be put to use.

In 1990 Karen's granddaughter was born to Karen's son Randy and his wife Melinda. Karen and Dave took an active part in their granddaughter's life, encouraging Randy to drop little Caroline off for a weekend as often as possible. Caroline's brother Ron arrived in 1992. Karen turned 50 that year and kept very busy, running her home, working full-time, and really enjoying her two grandchildren on many weekends.

Seven years sped by.

Chapter 5

Diagnosis

Karen had never had a large appetite. When she became engrossed in working on a financial plan for a client, it was not uncommon for her to skip lunch. At home she could start a project shortly after rising, only to realize at 5 or 6 p.m. that she hadn't eaten all day. In spite of eating so little, in 1999 she realized she was gaining weight. At first she noticed the waistbands on her clothing were snug. She had digestive problems, passing gas at embarrassing moments while at work or church. She was unable to shake the feeling that something was very wrong, so she contacted her family doctor.

The diagnosis was Hepatitis C. Karen remembered hearing she had contracted hepatitis thirteen years earlier when she had Hodgkin's disease, when she had received those transfusions of platelets. Now it seemed clear that the infected blood was almost certainly the cause of the Hepatitis C diagnosis.

At age 57 Karen found herself on another chronic disease management path. It was the advice of Karen's doctors to follow a strict low-sodium, low-protein, and no-alcohol regimen. She was told not to take any prescription or over-the-counter medicines unless they were prescribed by or approved by her doctor. She was told to increase her energy through regular exercise.[3] Karen was told she would be required to have routine blood tests so she and her doctors would know how well her liver was working.

Karen's doctors began to talk to her about the possibility of an organ transplant. Initially, the idea was to keep her liver as long as possible. This advice implied a grim reality: As the disease continued to get worse, it could cause her liver to stop working. In that event a liver transplant would be the only way to extend her life.[4]

Karen consulted the Internet and began the process of becoming educated about liver disease. Hepatitis C is a blood-borne virus.[5] It enters a person's bloodstream, perhaps from a blood transfusion or through the use of shared needles[6], and then passes to the liver. It is an infection that does not respond to a person's immune system.[7] (Hodgkin's disease, incidentally, is an immune system disease; Karen's immune system had been compromised in 1986.)

The hepatitis infection attacks liver cells. While a person's immune system tries to fight the Hepatitis C Virus, the person's liver becomes inflamed. Quite simply, hepatitis is the medical term for an inflamed liver. At the same time the inflammation is happening, the virus keeps reproducing.[8]

The liver is an amazing three-pound organ. It can heal and replace portions of itself (to a certain degree). If one section is diseased or injured, other liver cells can take on the chores of the damaged ones.[9]

A person with Hepatitis C Virus may have no symptoms.[10] Some symptoms of the disease, such as fatigue or muscular aches, may be associated with other illnesses or concerns, such as the flu, or a stressful job or stressful time in a person's life. Over time, the number of diseased liver cells and inflammation of the liver actually causes scarring, which is irreversible. This scarring of the liver is called cirrhosis.[11] So even while the liver is waging war with the infection, the Hepatitis C Virus almost always "wins." Some patients can be treated with "interferon drugs."[12] By the time Karen was diagnosed in 1999 with Hepatitis C, her disease was already too far advanced for interferon treatments to be effective.

Some of the symptoms a person with Hepatitis C may experience, in addition to fatigue and muscle aches, are low fever, nausea and vomiting, loss of appetite, and stomach pain. Karen had been receiving chemotherapy treatments back in 1986 when she acquired the Hepatitis C Virus in platelets, so both she and her doctors would have attributed those symptoms and her related discomfort to chemotherapy and its side effects.

Clearly, the Hepatitis C Virus had a chance to enter Karen's bloodstream, attack her liver, and cause scarring, all undetected, for a very long time.

Shortly after her diagnosis, Karen began to do research on facilities that have liver transplant programs and that were not too far from her home. She examined surgery success rates as well as transplant patient survival rates following transplant surgery. In June 1999 Dave accompanied Karen to a six-day series of appointments at a facility Karen had chosen, Baylor University Medical Center at Dallas, Texas. She had made arrangements with her local physician, who had given her a referral to be seen. During that week, Karen's condition was thoroughly evaluated.

At the end of the medical assessment, she was officially placed for the first time on the national transplant waiting list. Over time she became more familiar with how organs become available by reading about both the United Network for Organ Sharing (UNOS) and the Organ Procurement and Transplantation Network (OPTN) that UNOS, a non-profit charitable organization, operates under federal contract.[13]

In the early part of 1999 Dave and Karen had started planning a summertime family reunion for the King side of the family. However, all plans for the reunion at their home had to be cancelled after her evaluation by the transplant team at Baylor. Instead, Dave traveled by himself to west Texas for a school reunion and to Green Valley, Arizona for a visit with his cousins. His trip was the first of several that led to a realization for the two of them. They decided to sell their home in Mississippi and move back to Arizona.

In a Christmas letter in December 1999, Karen wrote she was "experiencing deterioration of muscle tissue and severe joint pain, which impedes the ability to do some daily activities like getting down on the floor [and back up again], reaching over my head to do my hair, or dress, or open things with my hands."

Paul and I visited Karen and her family for Thanksgiving that year, and witnessed some of these changes. When she got down on hands and knees to find a serving dish at the back of a kitchen cabinet, she needed both Dave and Paul to help her get back to her feet again. We made jokes about needing the help of the men to open jars of olives and pickles.

Karen had to make many adjustments for her deteriorating condition. She complained about having to "go at a snail's pace." She was not as independent as she had been. And she was still gaining weight. Instead of the hourglass figure and tiny waist of the past, her shape was beginning to look more like a pear. A side effect of liver disease is an accumulation of fluid in the abdomen. Even though Karen still ate very little, she began wearing Extra Large sweaters that reached nearly to her knees (and which covered up her expanding tummy and hips).

She also made adjustments for her work. She was advised not to drive a car, in part because her doctors didn't want her to be alone in a car for her lengthy commute. The computer guru from Karen's financial planning firm set up a computer in Karen's home, allowing her to connect to the databases and files she needed to continue writing plans for clients. Dave was retired by this time, but worked part-time at jobs near their home. He gladly drove Karen to the office once a week for meetings. He became the chief cook, laundry-man, and housekeeper in addition to chauffeur while Karen worked in her office at home.

In 2002 Dave had a mild heart attack and a pacemaker implanted. Karen and Dave's roles were reversed. With this big change, Dave's health issues became Karen's primary focus. Dave also learned he had emphysema, due no doubt to his nicotine addiction; he had smoked cigarettes all his life. Although he tried repeatedly to quit, he was never able to "put them down," as he so often called it.

In another one of her King family Christmas letters to others and to us, Karen wrote that she and Dave had begun joking about how their retirement years had turned out. Instead of taking numerous trips as they had dreamed, their health issues prevented them from doing many of the things they would have liked. Paul and I often remarked that Karen's health issues and Dave's health issues were both very serious. We wondered which one was going to take care of the other one, and the answer to that question kept changing. As she had done when Karen had Hodgkin's disease, Penny answered a call for help once again, this time from Karen. Penny arrived in Mississippi to help her sister take care of her brother-in-law for an extended period.

Over time, Karen began the process of packing and preparing their house for sale. More time passed and various health issues were addressed. Finally in September 2004 after the house sold, Paul flew out from New Mexico to drive a moving truck west to his sister's new home in Green Valley, Arizona. As the moving truck rolled through New Mexico on a Friday afternoon, I joined the procession in my car. Karen was glad to get out of the cab of the truck and into the front seat of my car to ride with me! Our driving trip passed quickly. Karen talked nearly non-stop, filling me in on details about her numerous adventures with packing and holding garage sales prior to the move.

We all arrived safely, just in time for Karen and Dave to close on the new house. After a busy weekend of unloading and unpacking, Paul and I drove together back to our home in Alamogordo. We began to look forward to having Paul's sister and brother-in-law living closer to us. It would be a 6-hour drive between our homes.

However, we were very worried about Dave. He moved very slowly, sometimes used a cane, and had become very thin. He wasn't able to help with the work of moving at all; he was simply too weak and could barely catch his breath. He was glad to be in Arizona. He had told Karen months before that he wanted them to get settled before anything happened, health-wise, to either of them.

During the fall of 2004 Karen continued to summon her energy to get the new house settled. With the help of a friend, she painted the rooms in various colors, covering the "new house off white" paint that had been there. She slowly unpacked boxes. The activity seemed to be good for her, she said she felt stronger, and, although she still had a pear shape, she lost a little weight.

Karen continued to care for Dave. He made several trips to the hospital as his doctors tried to control his various medical conditions. Sadly, Dave was becoming more weak and frail. Lea visited her parents for Thanksgiving. The three of them took pictures and really enjoyed each other's company.

Dave went into the hospital again shortly after Thanksgiving. It didn't seem possible, but he lost more weight. He needed oxygen to help with his breathing. When pain management became the primary focus of treatment for Dave, Karen became very concerned. She was afraid she could not handle his care alone because at times he didn't recognize her, or couldn't grasp where he was. As Christmas approached, Dave was anxious to get out of the hospital and home for the holiday. Karen was torn; she wanted him home but knew he was extremely sick.

On the very day Karen brought him home from the hospital, Dave King passed away. It was December 23, 2004; he was 66. Paul and I rushed to Green Valley to be at his sister's side. Perhaps because it was Christmas, Karen kept her emotions under control. I never saw her cry and figured if she did, it would have been in the privacy of her room. I knew she was sad, but suspected there were also some feelings of relief. Dave's condition had given him excruciating pain and everyone wanted him to have a release from that pain. Paul and I were there to lend whatever support we could, simply by being there. Dave's cousin, Norma and her husband Harry became involved, too, and they insisted that the five of us go to a restaurant for a quiet Christmas dinner. At least no one had to cook.

So for several days, Karen handled her grief by keeping extremely busy, checking information on the computer, reading mail, making phone calls, and writing lists. She decided to have two services, one in her new city in Arizona and one in Mississippi, where the family had lived for nearly 25 years. She made arrangements to fly to Jackson, coordinating with her daughter and son. She called Penny, who once again rushed to her sister's aid. The two women met at the Dallas airport and then flew together to Jackson, where they stayed with Lea. Penny stayed close to Karen so she would not be alone at any time during that period.

Penny and Lea helped prepare the arrangements for the memorial service, which was held at the end of January in a church where Karen and Dave had been members. Randy, his children Caroline and Ron, and Randy's ex-wife, Melinda joined Karen, Lea and Penny for the service. The other service, which Paul and I attended, was held in Green Valley a week later.

Chapter 6

An Indomitable Woman

Karen was 62 years of age and a widow. It was 2005, and for the first few months of the year Karen tackled the challenge of putting Dave's affairs in order. Once again, her background in financial planning and insurance served her well.

Karen's mother passed away in April 2005. It was another sad time for the entire family, but especially so for Karen. Shortly after Dave's death she had begun planning a trip to visit her Mom, but received the phone call about her death before she was able to get there. Instead, Karen attended her mother's funeral.

After months of dealing with red tape, phone calls and numerous forms and letters, Karen decided it was time to do some traveling and visiting. Perhaps because of her own illness and also because of the two recent deaths, she seemed determined to get on with the business of living. She wrote in her Christmas letter later that year that it was "a year of travel to help get through my loss."

She drove by herself to California to visit an aunt in June. In July she invited her sister Penny to come visit. Together, they drove to Alamogordo to visit Paul and me. The two sisters drove north to Colorado to visit other family and friends, and returned to Alamogordo on their way back for a second visit with us.

While at our house, Karen announced that she was feeling pretty well and asked Paul and me if we wanted to go with her to England in a few months. She knew we had been to Europe before and are experienced travelers. Wasting no time, Paul and Karen sat down at a computer and made airline reservations for three of us; an 18-day trip was planned for November, about four months in the future.

In August and September, Karen made a series of appointments with doctors in Green Valley and Tucson to see how her liver was doing. As instructed years before, she knew she had to have regular blood tests. Her local endocrinologist told her that her liver disease had worsened. He referred her to a facility known for its transplant program, the Mayo Clinic.

Dave's cousin Norma became Karen's companion for trips to Phoenix. Although Norma and Karen had not spent a lot of time together before Karen's move to Green Valley the year before, Norma welcomed Karen with open arms. She said, "You were married to my cousin all those years, so to me, you're family!" Together the women learned and memorized the drive from southern Arizona to the various Mayo facilities in Phoenix, some 150 miles away.

Once the initial series of appointments was complete, Karen described for us the very thorough evaluation she had received. The Hepatitis C diagnosis was confirmed, and she was re-registered on the national transplant list, this time through the Mayo Clinic. The team at Mayo conducted its own series of tests, stating that the assessments done many years earlier at Baylor were outdated. At one of the Mayo visits, Karen had an ECG of the chest, a mammogram and a GYN appointment, to name a few. She met with someone in the psychology department. She was required to describe her views and feelings about the possibility of getting a liver from a deceased donor as an option, and said she understood that for a transplant patient to have a second chance it meant that someone else had died. She said she had given the notion a lot of thought since first being placed on a transplant list years earlier, and felt it was something she could handle.

At the end of September Paul and I went to Karen's home for a visit. We accompanied her to one of her Mayo appointments in Phoenix. She was scheduled for an ultrasound of her liver and a biopsy of the largest of several tumors that had been detected in her liver. Ultimately, the biopsy procedure had to be cancelled, so the team at Mayo was not able to confirm the status of the tumors that were in Karen's liver.

It was Paul's and my first introduction to the Mayo environment. It was unlike any other hospital we had ever visited. There is an air of professionalism as well as a genuine interest in every person that passes through the doors. We were very impressed the entire time we were there. Even the lobby is beautiful; it includes an open atrium and, at certain times of the day, volunteers play a piano. Karen asked Paul to become her Power of Attorney for Health Care and Mental Health Care. The Health Care Directive form was signed and witnessed at the Mayo Clinic Hospital.

Through the fall, still more appointments were scheduled. Karen had a CT scan of her chest. An upper endoscopy, using a thin scope with a light and camera at its tip, was performed. It was to allow a look at the upper digestive system and to look for any bleeding.[14] She saw a dermatology specialist. They did a specialized test to evaluate the motion and function of her heart. Finally, something called a Chemo-Embolization (injecting chemotherapy drugs right into the tumor area in her liver) was performed. It was supposed to shrink the largest of the tumors.

As the date for the European vacation approached, Karen talked excitedly with people at Mayo about her trip to England. Some of the staff indicated that they didn't think it was a good idea to take such a trip. However, Karen was determined that she was going to go. She obtained instructions about what to say and who to contact if she needed a doctor or emergency room visit while she was gone. However, she chose not to share the Mayo caution or any of their instructions with Paul and me. She knew she might not be alive in a year and did not want to miss the opportunity to see some sights in the United Kingdom. I'm not sure we would have been as eager to go on such a long trip out of the country had we known the folks at Mayo were against it. Regardless, Paul and I were very aware that we would have to keep an eye on Karen at all times.

The trip was a success, especially for Karen. Paul rented a car and generously drove his sister and me around many parts of England and Scotland. Paul and I changed our habit when it's just the two of us, abandoning our easy handling of our rolling suitcases and frequent walking tours of new places. Instead, we developed routines for our threesome; Paul or I carried Karen's suitcase for her. I helped her numerous times each day with her backpack purse. She was very heavy by this time, and was not as mobile or nimble as she had been in July when the trip was planned. She wore a pair of hiking boots and walked with a flat-footed, plodding gait. She brought her various medicines with her. Fortunately it was 2005, before airline restrictions on liquids were imposed.

Though Karen's activity level had decreased a lot even from the time we had last seen her, we encouraged her to walk short distances when we thought she could manage it. Often Paul dropped the two of us off, parked the car, and then walked several blocks to catch up to us. I instinctively knew I had to stay near Karen at all times. She was *not* comfortable in the colder weather. Her hands were weak and stiff; she often dropped things, and could not bend over to retrieve them.

One night we arrived in Morecambe, a beautiful seaside location in northern England. The car had been parked for the night, so we walked along the beach in the brisk November air to find something to eat. Both Karen and I ordered tuna fish, but it didn't agree with her at all. The next day she battled several bouts of intestinal distress and diarrhea. The proprietors of the Bed & Breakfast were so sweet; they brought toast and tea while Paul and I went out briefly to see some of the area sights.

When we all returned to our home in New Mexico, Karen went to bed. Jet lag and overseas travel is hard on anyone, but it was especially hard on her. We arrived home late on a Tuesday evening. On Wednesday I did some grocery shopping; Thursday was Thanksgiving Day. Karen got up and dressed in time for dinner in the middle of the day. She was extremely sluggish on Friday. We didn't learn until weeks later that she had miscalculated the number of days she would be gone from her home and had run out of her laxative that was critical in controlling toxins. She was suffering from her hepatic encephalopathy, so she was unable to tell us she could use an over-the-counter laxative once or twice in place of her Lactulose.

Observing her condition, Paul and I discussed Karen's situation in private. We agreed that she could not and should not drive herself home. We decided that I would drive Karen home in her car and Paul would follow in our car. She slept much of the way, which was unusual for her. She always said she was not "a nap person."

Paul and I returned home. When Paul called to check on Karen a few days later, she told him she was still spending a lot of time in bed. Living alone, she could follow whatever schedule she liked. It was nearly two weeks after returning from the trip to England, so Paul knew it wasn't jet lag still affecting Karen. He encouraged her to see a doctor and to get up and get out of the house at least once every day. He told her, "You have to keep your strength up." Karen promised she would push herself to go somewhere, even for a short while, each day.

At our home we could not know if Karen was taking her medications as prescribed. (We realized the intestinal upset episode in northern England was a blessing in disguise, as it really cleaned out toxins and ammonia from her body shortly before our flight home.) We also didn't know if Karen was exercising or walking short distances in order to stay mobile. In hindsight, maybe we shouldn't have taken the trip. But Karen was so determined. She even said, "No matter what happens in the future, I'm glad I went to Europe." The simple fact of the matter was that Karen didn't know what her future held, whether she would get *or survive* a liver transplant. She wanted to go to England in her lifetime and she had no regrets for going.

Paul continued to stay in touch with Karen by phone during the first part of December. It became clear to us that she wasn't managing very well on her own. Paul consulted with his sister Penny. Thanks to some very good luck and chance events, the two of them realized she could spend some time staying with their sister. Penny was an excellent choice because she had previous experience in the medical field as an Emergency Medical Technician and had worked in a hospital for more than ten years.

Answering the call once again to aid her sister, Penny arrived a few days before Christmas in 2005. Though she had been stubbornly resisting the need for help, Karen welcomed the company and soon realized how tough it had become to be living on her own. That winter, Penny tended to the house and many of the chores Karen had been unable to do for weeks.

Paul and I drove to Arizona for Christmas in 2005, and the three siblings celebrated the holiday together for the first time in more than 30 years! Karen made a fancy, decorated cake for dinner, which was held across town at Norma and Harry's home. It took her all day to make and frost the cake. In years gone by, it would have been about a two-hour job.

It was during the Christmas visit that I started to notice Karen's talkative personality was changing. She seemed content to let others carry on a conversation around her, as if it was too difficult to formulate sentences or to join in with thoughts of her own as she had done in the past.

As January 2006 began, Paul kept in touch with both his sisters. As part of her new, more quiet conversational style, Karen would usually say she was "pretty good," unwilling or unable to tell anyone how she was really feeling. By then it was too difficult to put her thoughts in order enough to describe what she was feeling physically. The rest of us did not know enough about signs and symptoms of things we should be watching out for.

Penny would tell Paul in private that Karen was sleeping a lot and exhibiting "memory problems," her phrase for the brain fog. She reported it was becoming more difficult for Karen to hold a conversation. Penny said she would watch her sister begin to do something, perhaps a task as simple as getting dressed, and get sidetracked over and over. Penny continually had to keep her focused on the task at hand with gentle reminders. Almost everything took more time for Karen to complete. In addition, Penny found it necessary to take over all the driving, housework and grocery shopping. She prepared most of their meals. Karen was still handling her own medications, so Penny wasn't able to learn, initially, what that regimen was or was supposed to be.

In the middle of the month Penny told us (after the fact) that Karen had taken it upon herself to increase her dosage of a diuretic she had on hand. Penny was shocked to learn Karen lost nearly forty pounds in a very short amount of time. Not surprisingly, at a doctor appointment in Tucson on January 16th Karen was told her electrolytes and potassium levels were not good. On the other hand, Karen had stopped taking her Lactulose to control toxins (resulting in two frightening trips to the Emergency Room in Tucson).

A few days after the first trip to the ER, Penny took Karen to a scheduled doctor appointment. Liver disease takes its toll on other parts of the body, and Karen was scheduled for an examination of her throat and esophagus. During an evaluation by endoscopy, she had some esophageal varices banded. "Varices" is the name given to certain blood vessels that were carrying more blood than normal, due to liver disease. The banding was done to tie off any blood leaks or ruptures that could occur due to high pressure and high volume of blood through those blood vessels.[15]

Karen also had a paracentesis done that day. This is a surgical removal, through a large needle, of "ascites," or fluid, from the abdomen. Several liters of fluid can be removed during such a procedure. Over the previous several years Karen's slim shape had changed. Her current pear shape became somewhat smaller after a paracentesis and the removal of so much fluid. But she always had a large swelling from just under her bust to below her hipbones.[16] The numerous medical procedures that day were tiring and difficult, so once again Karen retreated to her bed.

Karen did not care for exercise very much since she had gained so much weight. She'd said for years that she had lost a lot of strength in her legs, starting with her Hodgkin's disease in 1986. As a rule, she did not make exercise part of her daily routine. However, she had purchased a glider exercise machine that had helped her get her legs in shape prior to the European vacation. But by the time Penny came to live with her, Karen no longer had the strength and balance to step up on it and use it.

Similarly, none of us knew how critical it was for Karen to keep moving, even if she didn't feel like it and even if her muscles felt weak. None of us recalled then how well Karen had been able to tolerate a dramatic increase in activity when she had to pack boxes and prepare for her move in 2004.

Penny didn't know first-hand what exercise and/or activity instructions Karen had received from the staff at Mayo. Karen also did not care for the cooler weather (cooler to her, even though in Arizona it rarely gets very cold). It seemed it was easier to stay inside, play Solitaire, watch TV or watch movies. No one suggested Karen should relinquish control of her medications and Penny did not have much success monitoring of her sister's dosages.

Two conflicting forces were at work: Karen wanted to continue to be independent and to be in control; however, due to fluctuating toxin levels, her cognitive functioning was clearly below normal. As a result, it is likely that she could not recall when (or if) she had taken her prescription medicine. Penny knew how often Karen was *supposed to* take it and often asked Karen if she had taken her medicine as directed to keep her liver functioning and her toxin levels down. Like anyone in that situation, Karen could tell by the wording of the question being asked that the expected answer was "Yes." She routinely assured Penny that she *had taken her medicine*. Penny realized later Karen had not been telling her the truth or really didn't know whether she had taken the medication when Penny inquired about it.

We became aware much later that Dave's cousin Norma possibly knew some of Karen's instructions, having heard such things during various Mayo appointments throughout the fall of 2005 when she accompanied Karen to Phoenix. However, she didn't think to share this information with Penny (or Paul and me), and none of us thought to ask her. Norma probably thought Karen was taking care of these things herself. Norma also probably thought Karen was sharing the information with Penny, once she arrived on the scene.

We simply didn't know what questions to ask about instructions given to Karen by the doctors and other transplant team members at Mayo. At the time it seemed intrusive to be "grilling" Karen about her various medications and instructions. After all, Karen had been taking care of her liver disease on her own for nearly seven years. But we all should have been asking more questions, both of Karen and of her care team at Mayo. Norma, Penny, Paul and I *should have* been discussing Karen's condition, both in conversations with her and in conversations in private. A record-keeping system cataloguing all exercise or activity instructions, medications and dosages, would have kept everyone clear and on track during that time.

Chapter 7

Status 7

February 2006. During her life Karen had raised her family, completed college, and fought a successful battle against cancer. She had become an accomplished financial planner and a grandmother. When needed, despite living with liver disease, she had packed and moved from Mississippi to Arizona. With sadness and grace she had buried her husband and mother. She had managed her health for years after her Hepatitis C diagnosis.

Now in 2006, through a series of events related to her failing health, Karen found herself residing in a nursing home in Tucson, unable to walk. Even more incomprehensible was that Jack Kelly, an experienced professional at Mayo, was advising Penny, Paul, Lea, Randy and me to prepare for the worst. Her children were being advised to visit their mother. But Karen's children put their uncle and aunts off, saying they would wait and see about getting to Arizona for a visit.

The next appointments for Karen at Mayo were scheduled for February 28 through March 1. As that time drew nearer, Penny made a phone call to us in New Mexico. She described the drive from Tucson to Phoenix, the need to stay overnight in a hotel, and reminded us Karen's care had been handled for almost a month by the staff at the nursing home.

She described how Karen still depended on her a great deal, calling on her cell phone from the nursing home when, for example, she needed more water. It seemed Karen knew she wasn't supposed to drink the ice water that would appear on her bedside table, but couldn't remember to ask for some of the bottled water that was stored in her closet. So she would call Penny, who would have to explain that she should press her call button to get someone to get her a bottle of water, *instead of calling Penny.*

Karen was not herself.

Once again, Penny was exhausted. Even though her sister was residing elsewhere, she felt the weight of care twenty-four hours a day, seven days a week. It was obvious she absolutely did not know how she could manage Karen and a trip to Mayo on her own.

Paul and I drove to Green Valley on the evening of February 27, and spent some time with Penny at Karen's house.

The next day when Penny, Paul and I arrived at the nursing home in Tucson, Karen was waiting for us in a wheelchair. She looked so sick, slumped over, and perhaps asleep. She was wearing heavy sweaters and had numerous blankets on her to keep warm. It seemed her internal thermostat was broken because of the liver disease. One of us pushed Karen's wheelchair next to the car and set its brake.

Paul stood in front of Karen, with one of his feet between her two feet. He told her to reach up and clasp her hands around his neck. He bent and slowly pulled her to her feet. As I eased the wheelchair out of the way, Karen and Paul started a slow, circular step-step-step "dance" to move into position so she could sit in the front seat of the car. As Paul bent at the waist, still bearing most of her weight, Karen also bent at the waist to sit, and Paul lowered her into the car. We were grateful for Paul's strength. It was good that the car had a large door and a wide front seat. After Paul moved out of the way, I was able to bend and guide Karen's swollen legs into position for the ride ahead.

A little more than 2 hours later, we arrived in the Phoenix area. Paul asked Karen where the hotel was. There was no answer. It was a tough question for her. Most times it would have been her normal style to respond immediately. It took her a while to remember landmarks and street names. Finally we found the right place. Paul left us in the parked car and went inside. Fortunately, it was a hotel that often accommodated Mayo patients as its guests, and there was a wheelchair inside the front door. Otherwise, I don't know how we would have gotten Karen inside. After another rendition of the step-step dance, this time in reverse, and pushing Karen through the doors, we all arrived in the hotel lobby. Karen and Penny checked into their room while Paul and I checked into ours.

A typical round of appointments at Mayo begins with fasting blood tests, and that next day was no different. We were up and out early in the morning. The patient has to check in at each department. One of us pushed Karen in still another wheelchair, which was available at the front door at Mayo Hospital. I watched as Penny spoke for her sister, answering for her when the lab technician or others asked questions such as, "What is your birth date?" "What is your Social Security Number?" "May I make a copy of your insurance card?" or "What is your address?" Penny had Karen's important insurance cards and a sheet of paper with all her information on it. It was just too much for Karen to manage her paperwork or to answer those simple questions. Instead, she looked at Penny as she spoke, and nodded in agreement when Penny gave the correct information. The talkative woman I had met twenty years earlier had all but disappeared.

Although we had spoken numerous times by phone, February 28, 2006 was the first day Paul and I met Jack Kelly, R.N. His business card described him as a "Liver Transplant Coordinator." After her many phone calls to Jack, Penny really felt she and Jack already knew each other, and greeted each other warmly. We met with Jack, who asked Karen a number of questions and reviewed the lab results. Once again, Penny provided details when Karen could not manage an answer. When Jack was finished, we all went into an exam room to wait for Dr. Evelyn Clarke, whose business card read, "Transplantation Medicine, and Gastroenterology & Hepatology."

We were told Karen's MELD score was 22. MELD stands for Model for End-Stage Liver Disease. It is used for transplant candidates, and the scores indicate how urgently a patient needs a transplant. On that day, I didn't know whether a score of 22 was good or bad; if Karen had been assigned MELD scores that were higher or lower in the past, I also didn't know that. We should have asked, "How high does a MELD score typically need to be for a patient to rise to the top of the waiting list?" But we didn't do that. We were trying to concentrate on the information we were being given.

The next thing we heard was that Karen's status was being changed to Status 7, which meant she had been "deactivated." She could not have transplant surgery at this time because of the clot that had been found earlier in February. It meant that if a liver (one which might be a match for her) became available the next day, she was *not eligible* to be chosen for surgery.

Then we were told Karen would not get a liver if she could not get up and get walking.

Dr. Clarke told Karen, "I see patients like you all the time. You are going to get worse before you get better. You are going to feel weak and lethargic. You need to get up and walk anyway. The stronger you are before you go into transplant surgery, the better and faster you will recover after the surgery." It was beginning to dawn on us that a patient needs a high MELD score. We later learned that MELD scores go as high as 40. Each person is assigned a MELD score, and it can change.

> "The Model for End-Stage Liver Disease (MELD) is a numerical scale, ranging from 6 (less ill) to 40 (gravely ill), used for liver transplant candidates age 12 and older. It gives each person a 'score' (number) based on how urgently he or she needs a liver transplant within the next three months. The number is calculated by a formula using three routine lab test results: Bilyrubin, which measures how effectively the liver excretes bile; INR (prothrombin time), which measures the liver's ability to make blood clotting factors; and creatinine, which measures kidney function. (Impaired kidney function is often associated with severe liver disease.) The only priority exception to MELD is a category known as Status 1. Status 1 patients have acute (sudden and severe onset) liver failure and a life expectancy of hours to a few days without transplant. All other liver candidates age 12 and older are prioritized by the MELD system. A patient's score may go up or down over time depending on the status of his or her liver disease. Most candidates will have their MELD score assessed a number of times while they are on a waiting list. This will help ensure that donated livers go to the patients in greatest need at that moment."[17]

Author's note: As far as I know, the designations Status 2 through Status 6 are no longer used and the MELD score/system has replaced those five Status levels previously used.

Karen was again slumped over in the wheelchair, and I wasn't sure how much she heard or understood. Dr. Clarke told us that they would prefer Karen to be in a nursing home in Phoenix so that she (and others at Mayo) could direct all of Karen's care. Karen was told she was going to be seen again on March 22, 2006, about three weeks later. Penny, Paul and I had discussed the night before how sick Karen had become. Among ourselves, we had wondered if perhaps Karen should be hospitalized. When we asked Dr. Clarke about this, we were told there was no medical reason to admit her. In other words there was nothing that couldn't be done elsewhere.

We had just heard Karen was going to get *worse*! I was in shock. We could barely care for her. It was an incomprehensible blow that, as sick as she was, Karen was not sick enough to be in a hospital but also not eligible for a transplant. What a horrible situation!

Paul said that when he glanced at Dr. Clarke as she left the room, there were tears in her eyes.

In retrospect, I wish Penny, Paul and I could have known to engage Jack Kelly and Dr. Clarke in more conversation. I wish we could have asked, "Aside from getting Karen walking, what are the other two or three things we should concentrate on most?" I wished we had asked for advice about caring for someone who cannot walk, since we were not learning much from the care she was receiving at the nursing home. We didn't seem to be able to focus on the "what's next" aspects of Karen's care. Instead, we heard what the Mayo nurse and doctor said in the moment and went away trying to absorb what we had heard.

Somehow, the four of us managed to get through the rest of the day. We went somewhere for supper and made a quick trip to a pharmacy for some adult diapers for Karen. Penny and I assisted Karen into the bathroom at the hotel. Karen didn't think to talk about the fact that she had been on constant bed-rest, and I didn't think to ask how she had been handling bathroom business in the previous days. Penny didn't mention a thing; perhaps she thought it was a good idea for Karen *to try* to walk and use the restroom.

Once again, we were not communicating. I've always thought it is rude to talk about a patient, in this case my sister-in-law, as if she were not in the room. But Penny and I should have been discussing a plan for the trip to the bathroom. We should have asked Karen what she could manage, based on recent events.

Anyway, we got Karen *into* the bathroom. We couldn't lift her up from the toilet, and I didn't think to try to have her clasp her hands around my neck as Paul had done. Since the bathroom was not equipped with bars, Karen had nothing to hold onto or use to push up with her arms. Her leg muscles were too weak to do the job of pushing her to a standing position. Penny had to step away, as her back was bothering her.

Somehow I assisted Karen with a slow, careful slither to the floor. Penny and I helped Karen get dressed on the floor; then Paul came in and first dragged and then lifted Karen up to the bed. From then on, Penny changed and cleaned her sister on the bed in the hotel room instead of going to the toilet. Each day was a huge challenge for Karen. Each day was a huge responsibility for Penny as her caregiver. Since we had not received information early on about how the disease might progress or what to expect, at every turn caring for Karen was a "trial and error" proposition.

During that night Karen decided it was time to get up and get walking. She _had_ heard what Dr. Clarke had said! When she tried to walk a few steps to the bathroom, however, her legs gave out, she hit her head on the wall, and she crumbled to the floor. Her leg muscles were powerless after nearly three weeks in bed, and her reasoning was addled, not allowing her to remember the bathroom incident the evening before or to anticipate probable consequences since she was still not strong enough to walk on her own. Karen tried to lift herself to the bed. When that failed, she woke her sister.

"Just hand me a pillow and cover me with a blanket; I can sleep on the floor," Karen said. Penny had learned at the house that she could not lift Karen, who by then weighed nearly 200 pounds. She handed Karen the blanket and pillows. They waited a few hours until morning, and Penny called their brother in the hotel room down the hall. Paul gently scolded Karen for getting up in the middle of the night.

"What were you thinking?" he asked. Karen agreed she wasn't in any shape to do any more walking. For the second time in fewer than

12 hours, Paul carefully lifted Karen from the floor to the bed, excused himself, and allowed Penny and me to get her cleaned up and dressed for the day. Paul mumbled his concern about seeing Karen's legs or other unclothed body parts. Karen quipped, "Don't worry—I lost all concern about that sort of thing a long time ago!"

While at breakfast in the hotel lobby, Karen received a call on her cell phone. It was the scheduling staff at Mayo, directing her to have another test, a CT (Computerized Tomography) scan, at 1:30 that afternoon. Our trip back to Tucson would be delayed by more than half a day. Late that afternoon, we dropped Karen off in Tucson and Penny returned to Green Valley. Paul and I drove home to New Mexico, arriving the next morning just before 2 a.m.

Chapter 8

Moving to Scottsdale

Over the next several days, Penny, Paul and I discussed Dr. Clarke's request. We were adapting to the needs of the time; there were so many problems to solve each day. There were issues with the nursing home and issues with the medical community. There were decisions to be made about where Karen was going to reside and receive care. There was red tape at every turn. We learned to focus on solutions and to keep our momentum up. We had to "let go" of the problem of the day before or the week before and put all our energy and attention on the issue at hand.

Since Penny was still visiting Karen daily and Paul had his business to run, I volunteered to make several phone calls to learn about facilities in the Phoenix area near Mayo that could accept Karen as a new patient. After many calls and coordination with Jack Kelly, I was referred to a social worker at Mayo. The social worker asked why I was calling on Karen's behalf instead of Penny, as she noted that her records showed her as Karen's primary contact person. I explained that I was Karen's sister-in-law, and that my husband Paul, Karen's brother, was Karen's Medical Power of Attorney.

She asked who Karen's caregiver was. Since I hesitated for a few seconds, she spent several minutes describing the tasks that would be required of a caregiver following transplant surgery. She said the person would have to live with the patient, administer a number of post-transplant medications, and keep records of all dosages and the time of day they were taken. The person would be required to take blood pressure and temperature readings and to do the cooking. She said the caregiver would have to drive the patient to all scheduled appointments at Mayo.

When the social worker completed her lengthy discussion of the duties of a caregiver and demanded for a second time to know if Karen had a caregiver, I replied that it was Penny. She said if there weren't a committed caregiver to be with Karen following a transplant operation, she would not be a candidate for transplant surgery.

I assured her that Karen would have a caregiver. I said that Paul and I were getting involved with Karen's affairs following the recent appointments we had attended with her at Mayo. I was surprised at how emphatic a point the woman was making about the need for a caregiver. On reflection, of course, it made sense. Karen's records showed she was a widow. Furthermore, I knew Karen had reached a point in her deteriorating condition where she could no longer live alone or even walk by herself. Her brain functioning had changed and she could not be depended upon to remember to take her medications. Certainly she would not be able to care for herself following major surgery.

The social worker stated that it was highly irregular for a transplant patient to be in a nursing home. While I was silently reeling from that statement, because I took it to be criticism about Karen's current situation and our family's handling of it, she went on to give me the names of three facilities with whom Mayo worked. Somehow I managed to write down the names, addresses and phone numbers she gave me. I thanked the social worker for her time. I guess she was doing a lot of her thinking out loud, and I realized if she had the names of three facilities, it must not be that "irregular" for a patient to spend some time in a nursing home. Besides, Dr. Clarke had suggested moving Karen to a nursing home in the area.

I began making phone calls. When I reached each one, I explained Karen's particular needs, namely that she needed to be in physical therapy and receive a lot of rehabilitation so she could qualify for a liver transplant. I explained that she was currently registered to be a transplant patient but that her condition was not good enough for her to be eligible for surgery. I described the muscle weakness that plagued her constantly and explained that she needed to be active and mobile anyway. I described the build-up of toxins when a person's liver isn't functioning properly, and the brain fog that typically resulted if she wasn't taking her medications properly. I noted that her medical care would continue to be directed by the doctors and staff at Mayo, and that the staff of the new nursing home would be asked to work closely with the team at Mayo.

After calling each of the three facilities, I received some very good news. A center we had driven past in Scottsdale had a vacancy and would be able to accept Karen on March 8th. The next step was to notify the nursing home in Tucson that Karen would be leaving. Once again Jack Kelly became involved. The reason written on Karen's release paperwork was *"At the request of family and at the direction of Mayo Clinic, Phoenix."*

It was obvious to Paul that Karen would again need his help moving from one facility to another. In addition, he had his copy of the Medical Power of Attorney. If there were any questions about why her brother was directing Karen's move, Paul could present that document. Besides, Karen was fairly lucid and on board with the change in location.

"If moving to Phoenix means getting regular care directed by the Mayo team, let's do it," she said. We drove over to Green Valley on March 7, and spent the night at Karen's house, visiting with Penny for the evening. Earlier that day Penny had left word at the Tucson center that Karen would be leaving the following morning so she could move to Scottsdale. She had packed Karen's belongings.

It got late and Paul said it was time for bed.

Chapter 9

Penny's Announcement

Just before preparing to turn in for the night, Penny said she had news. She said she needed to schedule some appointments with her doctors and was flying out of Tucson the next morning. She didn't elaborate very much at the time, but we knew she had undergone surgery on her spine the previous April. She had suffered some complications during surgery and was not healing as hoped.

We learned later that caring for Karen had taken its toll. The constant stress had exacerbated Penny's ulcerative colitis. When Karen fell to the floor after falling asleep in her soup, Penny had seriously re-injured her back trying to help her up. She hadn't complained. She was trying valiantly to take care of her sister. She had moved to Green Valley willing to do whatever it took to get Karen through her ordeal, but Penny's own medical conditions had become critical. It was time for her to see to her own health issues, which could no longer be ignored.

Penny promised she would be back in a few weeks. She also pointed out to us that Karen was about to be moved to a location more than 150 miles away from the house. Daily visits would no longer be possible. Penny told us she had arranged for a ride to the airport the next morning with Norma, which would free Paul and me to concentrate on going to Tucson and later to Scottsdale with Karen.

Our all-consuming focus at the time was Karen. Paul and I were so intent on getting her move accomplished that we didn't pay much attention to what Penny was telling us about her own medical conditions, or the implications of her absence.

After saying goodbye and seeing Penny off to the airport with Norma very early on March 8, Paul called Karen. He reminded her to tell the staff we would be there to pick her up at 10:30.

But it was not to be.

We arrived just before 10:30 but Karen wasn't discharged until 1:30 p.m. She was given sixteen prescriptions to take with her. She had not been given any medicine or meals that day, since the staff had been told she was going to be discharged. In spite of all that, Karen was in a very good mood. After we took her to the car in a wheelchair, she cracked some jokes and enjoyed riding in the front seat and talking with Paul.

Following the 2-hour drive, we finally arrived at the new nursing home in Scottsdale. We saw to it that Karen was checked into her room late in the afternoon. She was exhausted, hungry, and needed a "restroom assist" from an orderly there. As soon as we saw that she was in her bedclothes and in her bed, we started our eight-hour drive home to New Mexico.

Over the next two days, Paul contacted Dr. Cho, the attending physician at the new place in Scottsdale. Paul explained he was Karen's agent under the Medical Power of Attorney. We thought Paul's instructions were clear and simple. He said Karen's ammonia and toxin levels needed to be kept down and her activity level needed to be kept up. He told Dr. Cho to leave word with all staff members involved with Karen's care that if her condition worsened, Mayo should be called and if so instructed, they should arrange for her to be transported to the Mayo Emergency Room or its Hospital.

Paul encouraged Dr. Cho to contact Jack Kelly directly for Jack's instructions about Karen's care. Dr. Cho did indeed call Jack, and then reported back to Paul that the two of them had talked at length. Both Paul and I were relieved that there was a strong, professional willingness on the part of both Dr. Cho and Jack Kelly to speak about the needs of the patient, and not get caught up in politics or titles of nurse or doctor. In the few weeks we had known Jack, Paul and I were impressed with both Jack's knowledge and competence in relating to patients and their families. Both Jack and Dr. Cho knew the care of the patient was the main thing and none of the rest of it mattered.

I believe much of the credit for this rare focus on the patient must go to Jack and the philosophy of the entire staff at Mayo. He is an experienced transplant coordinator working within an extraordinary organization. He was willing to share his knowledge with another person, Dr. Cho, who was joining Karen's care team, and to bring the doctor up to speed on what was critical for her on-going care. Similarly, Dr. Cho was an attentive and quick learner. He truly wanted to learn how to care for a transplant patient, and made it his business to become informed and act on the new information. Karen was not a typical nursing home resident in the final stages of life.

Paul is an accomplished business manager who demanded a high level of communication. He understood his role for his sister to be one of an on-going education process, and while he (and I) did not know it all yet, we knew enough. We knew Karen needed specialized care to become stronger in order to be ready for a transplant. Her move to Scottsdale was an amazing example of how special people and various things fell into place, in just the right way, at just the right time for Karen.

Chapter 10

Mayo Magic

Paul called Jack Kelly to remind him Karen could be reached on her cell phone. Paul made sure Jack had our cell phone numbers, too. Jack told Paul he was impressed that the family arranged to move her so quickly. We learned it *can* take weeks or months to find a room for a patient in an extended care facility. We were thrilled to have accomplished Karen's move in just a few days. Paul told Jack that he and I would be Karen's primary contacts until further notice. Jack remarked how knowledgeable and helpful Penny had been as Karen's contact person up until that point.

In one of the conversations with Jack, he expressed *again* that he thought everyone in Karen's family needed to begin to prepare for the worst. Jack had begun discussing the need for family members to come visit in the middle of February; it was mid March and he was bringing the subject up again. He said that if the family members were planning to come visit, it should be soon. Paul continued to press his niece and nephew for those visits. We knew Randy and Lea had just lost their Dad a little more than a year earlier. We also recognized it is expensive to make travel arrangements, and not every organization is generous about granting time off. And we were quite sure Karen's children were scared.

As noted, in her new room, Karen had her cell phone to use. In fact it was her only way to have any contact with us. We weren't sure if she kept it by her bedside. We didn't know when her physical therapy sessions were held, or when her mealtimes were scheduled. Sometimes

Karen would forget to plug the phone into its charger, so a call from us would not go through. For several days we tried to call Karen numerous times, but were unable to reach her. Each night Paul and I went to bed hoping that Karen was in the right place, and that Dr. Cho and the staff was monitoring her needs carefully.

On Wednesday, March 15, just a week after we moved Karen, we were finally able to reach her by phone. She slurred her words. She would begin speaking, but trail off and not finish her sentence. Since it was dinnertime, we asked how the food was at the new facility.

"It's hard to eat in bed," she replied. We asked if she had been going to the dining room for her other meals, and she said, "I haven't been going to the dining room, I'd rather stay in bed." Oh, oh. Paul and I suspected her toxin levels were elevated and the vicious cycle of brain fog, sluggishness, and muscle weakness was back. Karen admitted she had been sleeping a lot.

We began to realize Karen wasn't able to ask for the things she needed, such as help with taking a walk. We were pretty sure she wouldn't ask for her medicine; she didn't like the diarrhea it caused. We wondered if she remembered Dr. Clarke's advice that she was going to feel bad but that she should get up and get moving anyway. Karen didn't seem to have the clarity to realize she should be going to the dining room for her meals, and take the opportunity to get some exercise. It was a kind of logical thinking, that is, "if I go for a short walk, maybe I'll feel better" that seemed to be lost in the encephalopathy or "brain fog" that was a side effect of liver disease. She seemed to be in another downward spiral where it was simply easier to do nothing.

Early the next morning Paul called Dr. Cho, who then examined Karen. He called Paul back. He wanted to be sure about Paul's instructions to contact the folks at Mayo. Paul said, "Absolutely, call Jack Kelly and coordinate with him."

Karen was transported to the Mayo Emergency Room that day at the direction of Dr. Cho and with help for her arrival at the ER from Jack. Due to the encephalopathy, Karen was given numerous doses of Lactulose, and in time, her toxin levels came down. A paracentesis was also performed, removing fluid that had built up in her abdomen since that same procedure had been performed on January 25 (seven weeks earlier). When Karen was lying still as instructed after her paracentesis, she felt something cool on her side. When she touched the cold, wet spot, she wondered how she could possibly have gotten wet there. Then she looked at her hand and discovered it was blood!

The large needle inserted in her abdomen had also nicked a blood vessel. She called for help and the bleeding was stopped very quickly. However, there was enough concern in the ER that a decision was made to admit her. Normally, the routine would have been to send the patient home, or in Karen's case, back to the nursing home.

The admission to the hospital turned out to be a lucky break for Karen. While there, she received enough medication to reduce her toxin levels and keep them low, so much so that she was able to borrow someone's cell phone and dial our home phone number from memory! Karen said she was concerned about *us*, concerned that *we* didn't know where she was or what had happened. (Of course we didn't tell her about the many calls we had made to or received from both Dr. Cho and Jack Kelly.)

Because the fluid had been drained from her abdomen, relieving pressure, and removing several pounds of fluid, Karen said she was able to move around better and seemed to have more energy. When that much fluid is removed, I thought later, it must feel like being able to remove a 10-pound bowling ball that was strapped to the front of your body. Platelets and albumin were given intravenously to aid her system with functions her liver was no longer performing well (or at all).

When I had been researching extended care facilities in the Scottsdale area earlier in March, I had been given the name of Ted Dailey, the Director of the Arizona Transplant House. I learned the Transplant House is a residential facility where transplant patients and their caregivers can stay during the weeks following transplant. It's considered necessary to be in the area near Mayo because transplant patients need to be followed (that is, seen) by doctors and others for several weeks after surgery, as the Mayo social worker had explained to me. I'd been told it might be a place where Paul and I could stay when we were in the area, depending, of course, on availability.

On Friday, before the close of business, Paul called Ted and told him about his sister. Ted looked for and found Karen's name on a transplant patient waiting list. He assured Paul we were eligible to stay there since we were Karen's primary contacts. Better still, Ted advised us he had a small room we could use for three nights, March 18-20,

2006. The Transplant House operates on a much-reduced fee schedule, so it sounded like a good deal to us. In addition, I was interested in seeing the place where transplant patients often stayed.

Paul and I drove to Phoenix once again on Saturday, March 18th. When Jack had called to give us a progress report on Friday morning, he reminded us that Karen's status was "deactivated." He repeated that in order for her to get reactivated, the blood clot situation was going to have to be resolved and her overall strength was going to have to get better. Paul and I were aware Karen's next scheduled appointments were coming up in a few days, on March 22. So I packed enough clothing for a full week.

We wanted to see Karen with our own eyes. Her trip to the Mayo ER and subsequent admission to the Mayo hospital was a concern to us. Living through the numerous medical crises was like being on an emotional roller coaster. We were worried that she had slipped into the current crisis in just a few days, but we also wanted to see her while she was sounding so well. We wanted to enjoy the high spot after having endured some real low spots. She'd told us on the phone, "I feel great."

It was a long, hot ride from Alamogordo to Phoenix. So when we got to the hospital that Saturday, we only visited with Karen for a short time. Her thinking was clear. She talked about her growing realization that it was up to her to fight to get her strength back. She had a sparkle. Her mood was euphoric, having become a privileged patient in the unique Mayo atmosphere for the first time. It was so much different than other hospitals she had been in, and it seemed she could sense the difference. She had experienced an incredible turn-around from the previous Wednesday when she couldn't finish her sentences. For the first time in a long time, we had a "normal" conversation. She sounded logical and determined, which was music to our ears. We were buoyed by her mood when we left her. We had to hurry to check in at the Transplant House while a volunteer was still on duty.

Remarkable things happened to Karen while she was in the Mayo Hospital that weekend. Dr. Clarke visited Karen during her rounds. She got Karen up and walking. She left orders for the nurses to aid Karen in several more walks while she was in the hospital. Surely Dr. Clarke must have given Karen a pep talk, too. Mayo is an outstanding place, and Karen received extraordinary care that weekend. She had not been motivated to walk until Dr. Clarke showed her *and told her* she could. Karen told us later, "I'm never going to let myself get to the point of not being able to walk again." Dr. Clarke had restored her hope.

Karen was released from the hospital in the very late afternoon on Sunday, March 19th. When we arrived back at the nursing home, we learned Karen was going to have to be processed as if she were a new patient being admitted for the first time. We pointed out she had just been there on Thursday morning. We were told she had been gone more than 72 hours so they would have to start over with their admission paperwork. I asked about the paperwork on file from her March 8-16 stay. No go. We were told we had to begin again.

Inwardly groaning, the three of us answered the various questions. Paul and I knew the things to discuss. Karen was pretty sharp with her answers as well. Because of Karen's recent enthusiastic report to us about her hospital stay and session with Dr. Clarke, we knew she was supposed to be walking many times a day. While we were completing the admission process, the three of us repeatedly emphasized Karen's need for lots of regular activity in addition to physical therapy and other scheduled therapy sessions.

The next morning Paul and I met Dr. Cho. While I stayed with Karen, Paul had many more meetings. He met with the Physical Therapy Department head, the facility's Head Nurse, and the Charge Nurse for Karen's section. Paul left word for the dietician. Over and over he explained that his sister was a liver transplant candidate and not a terminally ill person. By the end of the day Paul said, "The Mayo hospital stay was the best thing that could have happened. Karen is better by far than she was last week. Thanks to all the discussions I've had with various people, the staff here seems to be really engaged for Karen."

On March 22, 2006 Karen was transported by van to her first appointment of the day at Mayo. I had arranged her transportation by telephone the previous week, since I didn't know at the time that Paul and I would also be in the area. We met Karen at the Mayo facility on Shea Boulevard in Scottsdale very early and took her to her lab appointment. Throughout the day Paul or I pushed Karen in a wheelchair to her various appointments. In contrast to how sick she was the previous month, she was able to give her own personal identification information when asked.

We learned some good news and some bad news that day. We were told the large tumor in Karen's liver had shrunk, according to the CT scan done on March 1, and that was good news. Karen's ammonia level was 278. I didn't know what a normal reading was, but that sounded alarmingly high. When I expressed my concern, we were told a patient with liver failure may have high readings but the most important thing to focus on was how she was actually functioning. We were advised not to pay so much attention to the numbers and to continue to pay attention to the preventative measure, which was regular use of the prescription laxative/toxin-reducing medication. We had been aware of episodes of encephalopathy off and on since the end of January, so this was good new information about how to deal with those symptoms.

We learned that the liver transplant selection committee met every Wednesday to review the various candidates who were waiting for a transplant. I thought it was good to know a review was done that often. We learned the names of the various liver transplant surgeons.

We met with Dr. Brown, whose specialty is Hepatology, or the study of the liver, gallbladder and pancreas, and the management of their disorders. He said his concern was the blood clotting. He asked the question, "Why is this happening?" He asked Karen if she'd had blood-clotting problems in the past. She hadn't. He drew a picture of the filter in the vein in Karen's abdomen, above the place where veins from both legs come in, discussing the possibility of having to prescribe an anti-coagulation drug, and the risk of the drug causing too much internal bleeding. Dr. Brown also discussed the risk of a clot going to Karen's lungs or heart.

"Sometimes a patient just has to roll the dice," Paul said. Without a word, the doctor seemed to agree Paul's comment was pretty insightful. Dr. Brown said he was going to order some additional blood/lab tests for something called a hypercoaguability panel, and to refer Karen to a hematologist, or blood specialist.

Dr. Brown repeated the fact (which we had first been told on February 28) that Karen's status was "deactivated." Karen reacted as if it was the first time she'd heard this information. Undoubtedly it was the first time she *understood* her status was deactivated, so it was very bad news for her. As soon as the doctor left the room, she broke down in tears, which I had not seen her do since she became so sick, not even in the days following Dave's death.

Paul and I hastened to explain her status was due to all the blood clot business, reminded her that the doctor had just called for some more tests, and that soon she would be seeing another specialist. While she pulled herself together, I babbled on about how the folks at Mayo keep analyzing a patient's various conditions and use the vast resources at their disposal to figure things out. It was true. I was reassuring Karen and I was reassuring myself, too.

At the end of the day, Paul volunteered to go to Karen's home in Green Valley and check on her mail. It had been two weeks since Penny had been there, and Karen was worried about bills that were waiting. We dropped Karen back at her room, and Paul and I drove south.

Over the next couple of days, Paul and I talked of little else besides Karen. We had seen how well she responded when we were able to visit every day. Although the staff at the new place seemed to be interested in learning about a patient with advanced liver disease, we thought we could help Karen more with her walking and activity level if we could be with her. We discussed Karen's first week there when she had not gotten enough attention and had slipped into another episode of encephalopathy. We knew from Jack's cautions that she could not recover from very many more (or perhaps any more) of these setbacks. "You've been worried about being with her since Penny announced she had to go home for a while," Paul said to me. So he made contact with Ted Dailey at the Arizona Transplant House.

Luck and good fortune smiled on us again. The same small room, number 6, which Paul and I had used the weekend before, was available. It was settled. Paul would go home to Alamogordo. I would use Karen's car and move into Room 6 again. I would become Karen's advocate and companion for a while as she regained some strength at the new rehab center.

When I arrived at the Arizona Transplant House I was given a key to my room and began to get my clothing unpacked. I would use the washer and dryer down the hall. That was a good thing; I only had enough clothes to last a week. Karen seemed happy to have someone who would drop in on her daily. Paul and I kept in touch by phone and through text-messages on our cell phones. In March, it was sunny and beautiful in Phoenix.

Chapter 11

Default Caregivers

Once I was settled, I decided to call Penny on her cell phone and give her an update. With all the activity of the previous couple of weeks, I realized we had not spoken at all! When I reached her, I told her about the new extended-care facility where Karen was staying and that I had gotten a small room at the Transplant House. When I finally ran out of updates, I asked her how she was doing, and how her visit in Texas (where one of her daughters lives) was going.

"I'm not in San Antonio," she said. "I'm with my son in North Carolina. I love it here, and I'm so glad I moved here."

"MOVED HERE?" my brain shouted!

I only heard a little of the words Penny spoke for a few minutes after that, I suppose about arriving there, and about her new granddaughter. I had assumed Penny would go to San Antonio when she flew out of Tucson, as that was where she had been living before and immediately following her own surgery. I thought she had bought a round-trip ticket, as she had said she'd be back to Arizona in a couple of weeks. I thought I would be filling in for her for a short time until she was able to return.

"Oh my God!" I thought. Just at the same time I had moved to Scottsdale, Penny was implying she was not coming back!

So I asked her about her plans to "see it through" with her sister, words she had used when she first moved in with Karen the previous December. Penny explained that her own health had become her first priority. She emphasized things had changed, and shared how impressed she'd been with how her son had found some doctors she could get in to see. She didn't comment on why she had not called during the previous two weeks, or if *or when* she was planning on telling Paul and me about the changes.

"Now that you've asked," she said in response to my inquiry about her plans, "I won't be coming back to care for Karen any more."

Even though Penny was concerned about her injured back, and her other medical problems, there was *joy* in her voice. Her burden had been lifted. It was obvious to me she had been busy getting settled. It was clearly a relief not to have to be thinking about her sister all the time.

"That's why she hasn't called," I thought.

It was also becoming clear the burden was falling to Paul and to me.

Although everything Penny said made sense for her health, I began to feel overwhelmed. Paul and I were being thrust into roles that we were unprepared for. Paul was not Karen's husband; I was not the sister with Emergency Medical Technician training. The enormity of the task ahead was difficult to absorb. When Penny and I prepared to hang up, I told her she should take good care of herself. Shortly after, we said good-bye.

Later that afternoon I visited Karen. Since it was the weekend, there were no therapy sessions. So we walked the halls at the rehab center. Sometimes Karen would push her empty wheelchair; sometimes I would push her in it. We sat in the sun for short periods. We explored the various sitting room areas. And we talked. It wasn't conversation that had any significance; it was more like friends discussing the day. It was sort of dreamlike for me, as only a part of my brain was concentrating on the conversation. Karen was in a good mood; she was still feeling buoyant from her hospital stay and the encouraging words she'd received from Dr. Clarke. Perhaps she was also enjoying my company.

I was realizing my offer to be Karen's companion while she was gaining strength could possibly be turning into something different. Penny was not coming back and I was there, possibly for the duration. I held back discussing my concerns with Karen that day; I felt she already had plenty of things to worry about during her illness and rehabilitation. And I thought maybe Paul should be the one to break the news to his sister that Penny was not coming back as originally planned.

As I settled into the routine of visiting Karen at the rehab center during the day and living at the Transplant House by myself at night, I realized it would be my home for an indeterminate amount of time. I had access to a computer, and decided to become a little more educated about Karen's condition, which is called ESLD or End Stage Liver Disease. I read an account on the Internet of a man who had *two* liver transplant operations. The first was followed by many complications; the second surgery went well and was successful.

One weekend I spent some time talking to a woman from California. She was living in Room 8. Actually, Room 8 was "the casita," a separate structure, which was probably the pool house when the home belonged to a family. (More on the Arizona Transplant House at Brusally Ranch later.) This woman's husband had a liver transplant on February 13, 2006, or nearly six weeks earlier. His pre-operative and post-operative issues, aside from liver failure, were related to how little he had been eating. His wife knew a lot about liver disease and the transplant process, so I was like a sponge soaking up information from her.

I reflected that Karen had to become reactivated again. The next hurdle was to try to figure out why she was having blood clots and how to treat that situation. I knew it was important to accompany Karen to the next appointment with a hematologist and find out what could be done about "the blood clot business", which was the term I had begun to use for that whole situation.

Meanwhile, Karen's world seemed to be shrinking. She became very focused on where things were in her room or whether an article of clothing had come back from the laundry. Her spirits seemed to sink again; the good mood following her hospital stay soon disappeared. She was consumed with her never-ending battle with diarrhea, which was the result of the laxative medication she had to take daily to keep her encephalopathy at bay and to keep her muscle weakness manageable. It made for such a horrible quality of life. Since she had been so weak for so long, especially following the forced bed-rest in Tucson, Karen still wasn't getting out of bed to use the bathroom on her own. So there were many times when she needed to be changed, and the staff at the nursing home wasn't always able to respond as timely as she would have liked. She wore adult briefs at all times. She talked about her accidents with me a lot, and I knew it was the part of her daily existence that was the most difficult. I was relieved Karen was in a facility where the staff was paid to do this kind of nursing. Not having the strength to get to a bathroom is a basic quality of life issue and I believed it was something Karen and her family should have been told about as a possible outcome. I believed she should have been encouraged to keep active enough so that it wouldn't have become an issue.

There was another characteristic of Karen's medication and related trips to the bathroom. She no longer seemed to have normal brain functioning to be able to anticipate the need for a trip to the bathroom. Using simple logic, I asked her how much time would pass after a dose of the medicine before she typically noticed the need "to go." It was a question she seemed incapable of answering. Instead, she repeatedly talked about what a surprise the accidents seemed to be to her. She related the notion that when the sensation hit there was no time and nothing she could do about it. She had become willing to accept not having control as an unpleasant part of her liver disease. She had become accustomed to being changed in bed rather than going into the bathroom by herself.

Karen no longer commented on what was happening in the world. I don't think she watched the evening news, and, while she didn't appear to have critical elevated toxin levels, her brain seemed too fuzzy to read a book or magazine. Her existence had become one of hanging on, just trying to get through each day.

One day I visited Karen in the late morning and noticed she was very groggy. I asked her a few questions so I could try to gauge if her ammonia or other toxin levels were high. She answered my questions and said she had been given a sleeping pill the night before. When I visited again at about 3:00 p.m. she was napping and didn't know I had arrived. She slept until suppertime and said she didn't feel like walking to the dining room. An orderly appeared and offered to push her in a wheelchair to the dining room; forty-five minutes later I walked to her table to see if she was ready to return to her room. She walked most of the way back, using the wheelchair for balance.

Karen's roommate had a dry, raspy cough. Before long, both Karen and I each had a cough, too. Every new or different problem seemed to be magnified in Karen's weakened condition. I began to think Karen shouldn't be in a semi-private room; she needed to be free of germs as much as possible. She saved a sample of the bloody stuff she was coughing up to show the doctor. Dr. Cho ordered a prescription cough medicine and a chest x-ray for Karen. He was very concerned about her, and his concern heightened my concern. It was one crisis after another.

Karen went to Physical Therapy when it was scheduled. One day, I found her in the hallway, walking back to her room. However, I learned it was the only time she got up to walk that day. For a while I couldn't figure out why she didn't get up and walk more, but realized it just didn't occur to her to do it.

When I got back to the Transplant House and my Room 6, I decided I should stay isolated from the others, due to my cough. The transplant patients living there were taking immunosuppressive drugs following their surgeries. I did not want to expose their compromised immune systems to a common cold bug. Then I decided to drive around and find a drug store, and once there I bought myself some cough suppressant medicine, which seemed to help.

Since I had Karen's checkbook and some other records of hers, another day I wrote out some checks to pay bills. She signed them when I brought them to her room. I followed up on some bills from her emergency room visits in Tucson by phoning the insurance company for her. While we were discussing all the issues related to her nursing home extended stay, Dr. Cho came in. Thankfully, he reported that Karen's chest x-ray was normal. Karen told him the cough medicine he had prescribed had helped.

When I realized we hadn't heard anything from the Mayo scheduling people, I called Jack Kelly. I had to leave a message for him, requesting the date and time of the hematology specialist appointment. Then I went to the office at the rehab center to inquire about a private room. The people in the business office told me they had a number of patients scheduled for release soon, and thought a private room would be available by the end of the week. Even though she was normally a very social person, I thought a private room would be so much better for Karen. Those two follow-up chores I did were things Karen didn't even think about and I realized were things she really needed help with.

Karen received a package from Lea. It included a "bed buddy" stuffed bear that Karen really liked and immediately named "Bailey." She told me Lea had given her bed buddies before when she'd been sick. She also received a package from Penny. It contained 14 little gifts; they were meant to fill the days until Penny's return to Arizona. I still didn't know exactly when Penny had changed her mind about coming back, and it didn't matter. I chose not to show Karen the note that came in the box; I simply followed the instructions and gave Karen a gift each day until they were all opened. Penny's changed plans were still not something I discussed with Karen.

Karen complained about the food she was getting, so one afternoon I brought her a crunchy chicken taco from a fast food restaurant. I'm sure it had too much sodium in it, but I thought she needed a treat. I left Karen early that day. As I left her, I reminded her to get up and walk again before bedtime. She was in her bed, under a sheet, without any drawers on, she said, because her bottom was so sore from going all the time. I knew her activity level was better, but she wasn't getting up to walk as often as I would have liked. I didn't know how much to push her, but I should have pushed her more. A dozen walks to the door of her room and back each day would have been better than just staying in bed or in a chair. Encouraging her to use the arms of the chair and to stand up, gain her balance, and then sit back down again, as a strength exercise, should have been repeated often. I just didn't know enough. I should have attended her physical therapy and occupational therapy sessions with her so I could see what kinds of exercises she was doing there so I could encourage her to repeat them in the evenings or on the weekends.

At about that time Karen asked me if I would be going home on the following weekend. I told her I thought I would stay another week, and go to the hematology doctor appointment with her. She said thank-you many times that day, and that meant a lot to me. I continued to hope I was doing some good.

Chapter 12

The Arizona Transplant House at Brusally Ranch

The following description of the Arizona Transplant House at Brusally Ranch* is taken verbatim from a marketing brochure that I picked up while I was living there.

<u>Rich in History:</u> In 1950 Ed and Ruth Tweed built Brusally Ranch on 160 acres in Scottsdale, Arizona. Tweed, who raised and bred hundreds of Arabian horses in the Arizona desert, was recognized as a leader in the industry and in Arizona. The Tweeds named the ranch Brusally by combining the names of their children, Bruce and Sally. In the 1990s, the Tweeds' daughter, Sally Tweed Groom, donated the property to Mayo Clinic Scottsdale. The home then was transformed into Arizona Transplant House at Brusally Ranch.

<u>A Home Away from Home:</u> Today the large Spanish-style home sits on six lush acres enhanced by large shady trees, colorful flowers, desert vistas, native fruit trees and plants. In addition to a serene environment, guests enjoy the use of a large kitchen and dining room, an out-door patio, benches located around the property and a putting green. The warm and inviting home is filled with fine woodwork, tile and ironwork, and each bedroom has a private bath and separate telephone extension. All bed and bath linens are provided and laundry facilities are onsite for guests' use. In addition to these amenities, the house has a large comfortable living room with a big screen television

where guests can gather to chat, relax or read. When you come to Arizona Transplant House, all you need to bring is your clothing, medication, food and transportation.

Guests Say It Best: Guests that have stayed at the house say the experience lifted their spirit; provided them with a peaceful and a meaningful setting in which to regroup and recover. In fact, those who have stayed at Arizona Transplant House say the powerful, yet calming atmosphere provided them with solace, as they found inspiration through the comforting words of others undergoing like experiences. In a word, it made a major difference in their healing—mind, body and spirit.

* Author's Note: The Brusally Ranch is no longer used to provide housing for patients. A new facility not far from the Mayo hospital in Phoenix was built and opened in June 2009. I'm sure the spirit of the ranch where I stayed lives on in the walls of the new facility, complete with a caring atmosphere provided by all involved in making housing available to those in need. (See www.aztransplanthouse.org and The Village at Mayo Clinic in Arizona.)

Arizona Transplant House Guests When I was There

My experience at the Arizona Transplant House is one I shall never forget. There were rules for everyone who stayed there, and staying there is a privilege. We were supposed to empty the dishwasher and maintain a germ-free environment, for example. We were polite in accommodating others when they needed to be cooking in the kitchen. We waited for the washing machine to become available. We knew to pitch in and just do a chore, such as taking the garbage out, if it needed to be done.

The rules actually inspired guests to be mature, nurturing, and caring. TV sets, which were located in common areas only, were shared. Without talking about it, all seemed to subscribe to the lofty goal of William J. Mayo, which I saw in the lobby at the hospital. The motto is, "The best interest of the patient is the only interest to be considered." William J. Mayo founded the first Mayo Clinic in Rochester, Minnesota with his brother, Charles H. Mayo and five other physicians.

The spirit of the House brought out the best behavior in everyone, in spite of the stress everyone had at the time.

There was some other conduct that seemed common at the Transplant House. When I arrived I met a woman who was there alone; her husband was still in the hospital following a bone-marrow transplant. When he arrived a couple of days later and his wife introduced us, I offered my hand in greeting. He was very focused on his need to avoid germs and said abruptly, "I'm not supposed to shake your hand." It was a learning experience for me and over time I learned that it was typical of many patients involved with life-threatening illness, surgery and transplant. Normal good manners and an ability to follow social conventions seemed to disappear. Instead, this focus of the patients on their own illness and their own needs was commonplace. The patients had been forced to consider death and their own mortality. They had been given a second chance, and they were determined not to squander it; they were determined to take extremely good care of themselves in the process. They were motivated by hope and the promise of the future, a long and healthy new life.

The Transplant House was nearly always fully booked; it became obvious to me there is a great need for reasonably priced housing. At Brusally Ranch, there were seven guest rooms and there were always seven fascinating stories. After a short period of time, I realized I didn't feel that I had much in common initially with the other guests there. I was seen as a caregiver, but my patient was living a few miles away at the nursing home. Karen was still awaiting a transplant. The others had already been through their surgery or some procedure(s), but Karen was still waiting to become "reactivated" and eligible for surgery. The majority of patients were there with his or her spouse; I was Karen's sister-in-law. I was often quizzed about Karen's immediate family members, probably both because of curiosity and concern. I felt their implied questions were, "Where are those people" and "Why aren't they here?"

On the other hand, I realized I could learn from the people there. They shared an immediate common bond with others who had been through similar, frightening experiences. They had each other to lean on as they were finding their way back to a "new normal" in their lives.

As noted, the couple from California was in a separate building on the other side of the putting green from the main house. Since he was still so sick when I arrived, I didn't meet him for several weeks. From talking to his wife, my sense was that the transplant itself went well. She said her husband was the sickest patient the transplant team had ever treated for a liver transplant, so he did not recover quickly. As his caregiver, his wife battled with her husband daily to get him to eat; she said he had not been eating much at all since the previous Thanksgiving, and it was March of the following year.

A couple from Douglas, Arizona was in Room 3. He had also received a liver transplant on December 13, 2005, but was still being seen regularly at Mayo more than three months later because his incisions were still not healed in two places. He was a joy to be with. He was always upbeat and seemed very healthy. He was someone I wanted Karen to meet because he was such an inspiration. I didn't have many opportunities to talk at length with him, and his wife, originally from Mexico, spoke very little English. Since I speak even less Spanish, she and I smiled a lot whenever her husband was not available to translate for us.

A couple from a Phoenix suburb was in Room 4. They had a number of adult children who came and helped out for a week or so at a time. I realized what an excellent idea that rotation was. Each grown child could check and see how their mom was doing and at the same time give their dad a hand with numerous caregiver tasks while there. The woman was a candidate for a bone marrow transplant. She was very sweet, although she seemed frail and weak.

A man, his wife, and her mother were in the only upstairs room, Room 5. The man had received both a liver transplant and a kidney transplant the year before and was back for his one-year checkup. His wife and I visited for a long time one day and it was encouraging to hear how well her patient was doing one year later. However, it was also difficult at the time to imagine Karen a year in the future; we were coping with her various issues on a day-by-day basis.

A woman was by herself in Room 7. She was a caregiver for her sister who'd had a liver transplant at the same time as the other two liver transplant patients did in December 2005, but was in the hospital at the time I moved in. In a way she and I had the most in common because her patient was away from the Transplant House, too.

Finally, I was in Room 6. I was impatient to get Karen to the stage where the other guests were, that is, out of surgery and recovering.

Because Karen was staying down the street at the nursing home, I had the experience of *not* needing to be with her twenty-four hours a day, seven days a week. But Paul and I had the stress and worry of her situation with us at all times. We communicated daily, both by telephone and by text messages on our cell phones. Both of us were (are) take-charge people. It was one of the most frustrating things I have ever been through not knowing what was going to happen next and, ultimately, how long it would be before Karen could have transplant surgery.

Would she be reactivated?

If Paul and I did not stay by her side, who else in her world would be able to go to Arizona and take care of her, even for a short time?

If we left Karen, what would others think of us?

Would Paul and I be able to live with ourselves if we walked away?

Did the people at the Transplant House and, more importantly, the people on the transplant team at Mayo believe Karen had an appropriate caregiver support system in place?

Was it up to Paul and me to tell others in Karen's family and circle of friends that if there weren't a caregiver in place, there would be no transplant? (In fact, it *was* up to us to tell family and friends what was going on, and we did a very poor job initially, of doing this.)

When Karen got her transplant, would there be volunteers to care for her then?

Would she respond like a "best-case scenario" case and be able to live on her own in six to eight weeks, or would she still be in Phoenix three or four months down the line, like some of the people I'd just met at the Transplant House?

If she required some live-in nursing assistance would her insurance cover it? Or could her budget manage it?

Would Paul and I continue to live apart for the sake of Karen's progress?

Would Paul and I be able to stay together after our own separation?

He'd said something in passing during that time that really startled me. "I hope this situation doesn't drive *us* apart," he said. I began to worry about my marriage. My offer to take care of Karen for a couple weeks had changed dramatically. Penny's health had suffered and she'd made the proper decision about not being able to come back. Paul and I had become caregivers by default, thrust into an excruciatingly difficult situation.

I had retired from my human resources career the previous summer. Paul had arranged things in his software company so that he and his business partner could provide customer support from anywhere in the country (and, in fact, with cell phones, anywhere in the world). So for the previous many months Paul and I had realized *our* dream of being free to travel. We had driven along the Alaska-Canada Highway to Alaska in August and had gone to Europe with Karen in November. Since the holidays were over and the weather in the southwest was spectacular, in the early part of the new year we were itching to get going again.

Instead we were in the middle of the medical emergency that was Karen's liver failure, and we had no choice but to muddle on as best we could. When I realized I'd been doing a lot of complaining to Paul, especially while I'd had my cough and cold, I subsequently realized that I needed to get "my game face" back on, for Karen, for Paul, for the other guests at the Transplant House, and for the Mayo transplant team. I realized I had to stay focused on the goal, which was to get Karen to and through a successful transplant.

Over the course of the next several days, Karen, Paul and I talked of little else but the subject of her on-going need for a caregiver. At first I hadn't wanted to break the news to Karen that Penny was not coming back. My observation of Karen's progress continued to be the one that had motivated me to volunteer to move to Phoenix in the first place, that is, that she did a lot better in terms of staying active and working on her own rehabilitation when someone was able to go and see her every day.

Paul pushed Karen to see the need for a caregiver as *her* problem, one she needed to solve. Karen suggested that she thought she could hang out at the nursing home on her own, and began to talk about the need for a companion *after* her transplant surgery. Clearly she didn't remember or acknowledge how she had slipped into episodes of encephalopathy too many times.

Paul and I told Karen about the emphatic and repeated conversations we'd had with Mayo people in the recent past on the subject of "if there is no caregiver, there will be no transplant." Paul and I had discussed Karen's need to get walking and to get her strength back. We had, in our minds definitely extended the need for a caregiver *for her* to include the time before transplant as well, so there would be less chance for her to slip into another downward spiral, possibly one from which she would not be able to recover. We had witnessed so many potentially life-threatening setbacks.

The three of us turned our attention to other possible candidates for the job of caregiver. Paul wanted Karen to call Lea and ask her to come live with her mother for a year or so. For whatever reason, Karen did not do that. Instead, she called a friend in the Phoenix area and her cousin Julie in California. Karen also called her friend Grace, whom she had known since both women's children were little.

I asked Karen about the many friends she had in Mississippi, since she had lived in that area for nearly 25 years. After she thought about that for a moment, she said, "But all those women are married, and they need to be with their husbands." What? I was angry and I was hurt. What about *my* need to be with *my* husband? I chalked her insensitivity up to her disease. I bit my tongue and forced myself not to make a comment.

It was hard to imagine what happens to other patients who are alone in the world. If someone doesn't have a spouse, a sibling, and/or grown children to help out, what do they do? I wondered if they would even make it past initial screening in a transplant program.

It came to my attention much later that Karen (with her husband's cousin Norma in tow) had told the Mayo people early in her evaluation process that she had caregivers lined up. On some form she had written both Norma's name and my name as the people in her life that would be there for her as her caregivers when needed. When I heard about it, I thought, "I guess Karen had my number." I was there. I was doing it; we were doing it. I wished she would have asked for our help instead of assuming we'd be there for her. Perhaps she thought she had asked Paul, and by extension, me, when she'd asked Paul to sign the Medical Power of Attorney.

Even though at the time there were other people including caregivers at the Transplant House to talk to, it didn't occur to me to ask for consolation about my feelings that perhaps I was being taken for granted by my sister-in-law, who was normally a caring person, and perhaps my relationship with my husband was in trouble.

Karen was finally moved to a private room in the nursing home. I realized I needed to focus on making sure the nurses and other staff members in her new unit were getting to know her and learning about her condition and particular needs. Educating them was critical and they needed to know what to watch for. In addition, I had to redouble my effort of making sure Karen got up and walked several times a day. She said it felt better when she did some walking. She used a wheelchair or walker to help with her balance. On Friday March 31st Norma, Harry and their son visited. Karen had in fact made some good progress following the Mayo hospital stay and her return to the nursing home on Sunday, March 19th.

It was gratifying to hear from Norma that she thought Karen had made *great* progress since the last time she had seen her in Tucson. She noted that Penny had shared how poor Karen's condition had been at the end of February. Norma was generous in her comments to Karen and in thanking me for my part in that progress. Karen basked in the praise; it was clear she needed and enjoyed encouragement. However, after they left, Karen reported to me that her calves hurt. I had to hope it was muscle pain from her busy day and not something else more serious.

After Karen was moved to her private room, it seemed the people at the nursing home lost track of her for a few days. She was moved on a Saturday; on the following Monday she was still not getting her food on time. That day, she didn't get her breakfast until 10 a.m. Unfortunately, I arrived after 10 a.m., so I wasn't able to track down her breakfast tray early in the morning. When lunch arrived, she said she wasn't hungry. She ate some vegetables. I left the room for a few minutes, and when I returned Karen was falling asleep in her chair. It didn't seem like encephalopathy; it seemed like exhaustion, another scary notion to think her body was wearing out. I asked at the unit desk if Dr. Cho was in the building and was told he was not in. I decided to stay with Karen through the lunch hour and I was glad I did.

Early that afternoon, the doctor came in. Karen told him about her latest crisis, which included nosebleeds and dark stool, an indication of some internal bleeding. She described having had her esophageal varices banded. Dr. Cho told us that when blood flows through a healthy liver, it picks up clotting proteins. But since her liver was so diseased, that was not happening. He said it also made her blood thin, and suspected that there was possibly some seeping going on somewhere. He ordered a hemoglobin test and asked Karen what her wishes were if the test came back with results not in the normal range.

Karen said, "I'll have to go to Mayo." I nodded in agreement.

After Dr. Cho left Karen's room, I called Jack Kelly, and told him about the latest symptoms and the test Dr. Cho had ordered. He said to keep him posted and cautioned me that Karen might have to come in so they could figure out where the blood was coming from. He told me to call again if the situation did not resolve itself in a day's time. As Dr. Cho had said, Karen was between a rock and a hard place, what with blood clots in her leg and bleeding from her nose and possibly elsewhere.

Karen's appointment with the hematologist was scheduled for the following day, April 5th. I worried she would not get there before she needed to be hospitalized again. It was another crisis, and the worry I had was daunting.

Chapter 13

Hurry Up and Wait

After the scare earlier in the week, Karen reported that her use of Neosporin in her nostrils and some warm air breathing treatments she had been given had helped. The bleeding from her nostrils had stopped. She also said the color of her stool was back to normal. All that was good news. What a relief.

But the appointment at Mayo with a blood specialist did not happen as scheduled. Karen got all ready for the trip. We went out to the Mayo facility located on Shea Boulevard in Scottsdale, and waited for the doctor listed on her itinerary (schedule). The nurse told Karen the doctor would need her to undress. Both Karen and I groaned when we heard that, as getting out of her clothing was no small feat with her expanded size and many layers she always wore to keep warm. I helped her with all the required tugging and stooping, and Karen did what she could. With Karen shivering and dressed only in a cotton gown, the doctor finally joined us.

He announced he was an oncologist, not a hematologist. He said we would have to notify the scheduling department to make a different appointment with a hematologist. What a mess. I wanted to shout and make a scene. But I had learned through years of dealing with personnel issues and outlandish employee emergencies how to keep still. This was certainly one of those times!

Many minutes later, fully dressed, Karen and I made our way out of the building. We learned from the scheduling people they had made an appointment with a Dr. Gossett, a hematologist, the next day. We

70

also learned Karen's next regular round of appointments would be on April 27, and would include routine fasting labs at 8 a.m. I realized it would be five weeks and one day since the previous blood work done on March 22. Other appointments would follow the lab session, namely one with a transplant surgeon, one with Jack Kelly, and one with Dr. Clarke. I was hopeful that an appointment with a transplant surgeon was a good sign.

Ted Dailey talked to me about possibly bringing Karen to the Arizona Transplant House. I had confided in him about Karen being a widow and that Paul was her brother and I was her sister-in-law. He mentioned caregivers who could be hired for $20 per hour and noted that such people typically have had background checks and were bonded, information I shared with Paul as we continued to explore options for Karen's care.

The day of the unneeded, messed up appointment with the oncologist, I brought Karen to meet Ted Dailey at the Arizona Transplant House and showed her around. Karen was able to walk through the office, through the small TV room, past (my) Room 6, through a hallway to the kitchen and dining room, take a turn around in the living room and walk all the way back out to the car. She did so with a walker, which Ted had allowed her to borrow when we arrived. She was tired when she eased into the front seat of the car, but I was impressed with how she pushed herself, probably to show Ted how much she had progressed.

On the flip side (and there always seemed to be a flip side), that afternoon Karen and I attended a Liver Transplant Support Group meeting. Karen introduced herself and announced she had moved to Arizona so she could be in Mayo's transplant program. I had *not* heard that information before that day. I paused to wonder why she hadn't moved closer to Phoenix; Green Valley is more than 150 miles away, much too far to commute and be seen as often as she needed to be seen. On the other hand, Karen had not been advised what the transplant process would involve, either.

I was jolted from my musing when I heard very clearly from the social worker that their ideal transplant candidate was not in a nursing home. She began speaking about the need for a committed caregiver that would be with the patient just before, during, and after transplant.

(I was pretty sure this was the same woman I had spoken to on the phone when I was researching nursing homes in the Phoenix area.) I later wondered how much the various players, had been talking about Karen's family situation, or Paul's and my roles as temporary and reluctant caregivers. I had not hidden the facts of Penny's departure or the lack of commitment from others that knew Karen.

The social worker asked every patient what his or her MELD score was. She looked at Karen and said that with a MELD score of 22 (and once Karen was re-activated), she would likely receive a liver sometime in the next six months. My ears and brain shut down after I heard that phrase, "six months." I couldn't imagine living in the Transplant House or with Karen from then, which was early April, until the following October! [18]

Knowing Karen would not be able to stay at the nursing home indefinitely, I re-focused and asked about other area housing. The support group leader and others said there were some one-bedroom apartments in the area for $650 per month (at that time, in 2006). Paul and I had been talking about what would become of Karen, as she was not in any condition to plan for herself. It wasn't feasible for her to continue to live at home and travel 300-miles (round trip) every time someone at Mayo needed to see her or run another test.

I thought it was interesting to learn in the support group meeting there was another woman who was also in a nursing home. She voiced her worries about insurance not covering her stay in the nursing facility as long as needed, which got my attention. I made a note to myself to check on Karen's coverage for all the days she had been in a nursing facility since the end of January. That woman's MELD score was lower than Karen's score, meaning she wasn't as likely to get a transplant as someone with a higher score.

Soon after the support group meeting ended, and when I returned to the Transplant House, Ted quizzed me pretty closely about Karen's situation, how long I thought I'd be staying around, whether Karen and her daughter got along well, whether her daughter would be coming to take care of her mom, whether Karen's son was available, right then (he wasn't), what about the other sister I'd mentioned (Penny), and did Karen have finances to afford a hired caregiver to help if members of the family couldn't play that critical role. Then it was clear to me everyone in the system wanted to know Karen *did have* a caregiver support system because without it, there would be no transplant. Again I wondered how much the various parties spoke to each other, or if it was simply a case of everyone "being on the same page" with concerns about Karen having a caregiver. I'm sure it is a common issue at a particular time as the patient's condition worsens and she also progresses toward becoming eligible for a transplant.

I knew the blood clot business had to be addressed and resolved first.

Karen and I arrived early for the appointment the next day, April 6th. Thankfully, she did not have to get undressed or change into a gown. Dr. Gossett studied Karen's case on the computer while we were there, making comments and asking questions as he went along. I took notes. He commented on Karen's Hodgkin's Disease/Stage III-B in 1986, the blood transfusions she had received (which likely gave her Hepatitis C), her splenectomy, the liver tumor that had been found the previous October, the Chemo-Embolization they had done at Mayo to shrink it, and the banding of varices. He talked about the blood clot found February 12, the filter inserted on February 19, her marital status and family status (widow, two children, two grandchildren, all out of state). He asked Karen what her profession had been when she worked (financial planner), and so on. He examined Karen. He told her to wear thigh-high pressure socks during the day or she would end up with a phlebitis problem that would not go away after transplant.

That was a phrase that caught my attention. "After transplant." It sounded so positive, so hopeful. It sounded like a "when" not an "if." I liked that.

The doctor said Karen's case was complicated. I thought to myself, "Understatement!" but once again I held my tongue. He said he was not particularly interested in knowing why she got some blood clots. He said her blood tests indicated she didn't need to be put on Coumadin. He reviewed Karen's recent supercoaguability tests.

Then he said he was pretty sure that Karen had Disseminated Intervascular Coagulation (DIC), or, in English, abnormalities in clotting, likely brought on by End Stage Liver Disease (ESLD). I gathered DIC is very complicated, and the upshot of the conversation was that Karen would have to be followed very carefully by the transplant team following transplant surgery.

He expressed some concern about the Greenfield filter that had been inserted in Karen's portal vein in February. He said he hoped it was a removable one. He noted that if it was not a removable filter, it could cause further problems.

Suddenly the doctor's musings really got Karen's attention. She told Dr. Gossett she was not activated on the transplant list. He dismissed her remark and made it clear he was strictly advising the transplant team about what was going on with her blood. He said it would not be his decision, but rather the transplant team's decision, about a transplant.

"A transplant will fix the DIC," Dr. Gossett told us.

It was the best thing we heard that day. *I was so encouraged by that doctor visit.* I wasn't sure I had written everything down properly in my notes, but I was optimistic that the hematology specialist's analysis could possibly be a turning point. The blood clot business, which had been going on for nearly two months, *seemed* to be getting resolved.

Dr. Gossett told Karen she'd hear back from Dr. Brown next, and the scheduling person we spoke to on our way out of the building also said she would get a follow-up phone call about an appointment with Dr. Brown. After we left, Karen said she was concerned about having to take Coumadin in the future. I reminded her that taking a drug for the rest of her life would be the least of her worries, and that we needed to get her to and through her transplant first.

To celebrate, we went shopping. I went into the store first, got a pushcart, and took it to Karen where she was still waiting in the car near the front door. Using the cart for balance, Karen walked in, saying she'd be looking at make-up. She chose some blush, hairspray, and later some ginger ale, hard candy, and some other items. I'd left her to park the car and stroll through the store to find her. Later that day I wished I'd have timed how long she was on her feet. I was pretty sure it was at least 30 minutes. Like the day before when she had met Ted, I was definitely impressed with how long she stood and walked. There was nothing like shopping to get her moving.

Continuing our celebration, we went to a fast food restaurant and sat in the sun. We talked about her options of where to live next. My preferred options were 1) The Arizona Transplant House, 2) an apartment, or 3) home in Green Valley. Karen was quiet. I was pretty sure all the talk about where she would go next was driving her crazy, too. But by some unspoken agreement, we didn't talk about our feelings. Perhaps we were afraid of the floodgates of tears and other emotions that might come rushing out.

After having left the Rehab Center at 8:30 that morning, we got back around 1:30 p.m. and Karen said "I had a very nice day."

I told her I did, too.

When I was driving back to my room that afternoon, Karen called. She said her physical therapist had told her she would be given assistance walking outdoors during the next week. She said once she had "passed that test" she would be able to be released.

At the Transplant House, I ran into Ted. He asked me about the doctor appointment. After hearing my description of the things Dr. Gossett had said, he agreed he thought it sounded encouraging. I told him I'd started talking to Karen about coming there to stay. He cautioned me Karen would have to be reactivated and he would have to know from the Transplant Team they thought it was a good idea for her to move there.

Then I called Paul to give him an update. He said he would probably drive over on the following Monday, April 10, 2006.

It was amazing how much things <u>seemed</u> to have changed that day: Cautious optimism.

Chapter 14

Time Passes

The next day I spent some time checking email before I went to see Karen. I was so pleased to read messages from a friend from home and from my sister, who wrote about how cute her grandson was at 8 months. It was great to hear about something from the rest of the world.

At the Transplant House the woman from Douglas prepared fish tacos for lunch, along with an amazing bread pudding dessert for everyone, so I stayed there until 2 pm. Karen was in a wheelchair in the sun when I got there. Before long she was discussing her numerous bathroom business mishaps, which was still the part of her daily routine and her care that concerned me the most. It wasn't that I couldn't provide that care for her; it was just that it was so hard for me to do it.

I longed to be a person who could handle anything, but I wasn't. Some of the personal care chores were intolerable for me and quite literally made me sick. It would be difficult, I believed, for anyone, whether a health care professional or not, to perform that chore many times a day. Karen never talked about being able to handle it on her own. It was frustrating to think her mental state, among other things, was preventing her from helping as much as she could. I knew her days at the extended care nursing facility were about to end.

Karen said that "from all Lea *didn't* say on the phone" the previous night, her daughter probably wouldn't be coming out to "help her" (as

Karen called it). She had recently started a new job and it would have been very difficult to get away.

Once again, I got depressed. I tried not to let Karen see it, but it wasn't long after that discussion that I excused myself and left her for the day. Paul called and I put all my worries on him, for example that I felt like I was "it" for the long haul and how disappointed I was in all the other members of the family. I told him Karen had just said that afternoon she never dreamed she was going to have to "go through all this."

"I always thought I would get registered on the transplant list, get a phone call that a liver was available, drive to Phoenix, and go in for surgery", she had said.

Paul reassured me that he and I would figure something out together. He added that it was going to be up to Karen to find someone and that it was *not* all on my shoulders. It wasn't the time that we had been involved with Karen's care after Penny left that was getting me down. Those days were done, and we had muddled through, focusing pretty well on issues as they came up. It was the unknown future that stretched out in front of us that really worried me.

So I went to a store. I told Paul I needed to change my focus for a while and get some shopping therapy of my own. Spending my time doing a normal, everyday thing like wandering through the store and buying two new t-shirts made me feel a little bit better.

When I got back to the Transplant House I met a man from Pinetop, Arizona, and his wife. He had a liver transplant on March 25, which was less than two weeks earlier, and looked amazing. I asked about his condition prior to surgery, and he said he was "sluggish" prior to transplant but was able to do mostly everything he wanted to do right up until the time he got his call. I didn't have the nerve to ask him about doses of Lactulose or diarrhea; perhaps that wasn't as much of an issue with him. But it seemed he basically *had done* his transplant in the fashion Karen had envisioned the process to be! Lucky guy. He even said he thought he'd be able to go home in about another week, or just 3 weeks after transplant. This was so uplifting to hear. I thought I really needed to get Karen over to the Transplant House again, to meet some liver transplant patients who were doing well.

What a day: another roller coaster ride with my emotions all over the place.

The guests at the house had changed again. A woman who needed a bone marrow transplant had recently come to the Transplant House from Illinois with her parents. Occasionally her grown son, who lived in the Phoenix area, also joined them and cooked dinner for all four of them. Another man from a Phoenix suburb who had received a heart transplant and his wife had also just moved in. Even though they lived nearby, he needed to be there for a short time while he was having numerous appointments at Mayo.

The other house members included the candidate for bone marrow and her husband along with their children who were, as previously described, taking turns to help with their mom and to give their dad a hand. So far two of their children had taken turns at being with their parents. It was a really good idea to have a team of people helping out. It was plain to see the husband was dedicated to being with his wife for the entire process, but not so good at cooking or other daily tasks. The others came in for short periods of time, observed how their mom was doing, took some of the chores and stress off their dad, then went home, resumed their busy lives, gained perspective, and "re-charged their batteries." A group of caregivers really sounded like a great way to go.

The other Transplant House guests were, as mentioned, the two men who had received new livers staying there with their wives, as well as the man who had just gotten a liver two weeks earlier and his wife from Pinetop, whom I'd just met. And there was me, for the time being alone, in Room 6.

It tickled me when patients introduced themselves. They would say, "Hi, I'm Fred. Heart." Or, "Hi, I'm Louise. Bone Marrow." It was such interesting and useful shorthand. The Transplant House accommodated lots of people. I realized again I was so lucky to have a room.

I continued to hope Karen would be reactivated and, of course, to get a liver soon. We had to be positive and hopeful. I prayed it wouldn't be four or five more months to wait. I recalled Karen had heard from Jack Kelly sometime in January and had called Paul and me to say she was Number 1 on the liver transplant list at that time.

There we were in April, three months later. Although she was getting her strength back, I knew her liver was getting worse all the time. And that was the worry and the cruel dilemma: Only the very sickest patients with the highest MELD scores would actually get a transplant. So at the same time a patient was trying to maintain reasonably "good" health, everyone also hoped she would be "bad" enough to get a transplant.

As planned, Paul spent 10 ½ hours in the car driving over from Alamogordo to Scottsdale on Monday, April 10, 2006. He took a route north to Socorro, New Mexico over to the Salt River Canyon, through Mesa, Arizona to Scottsdale. I forgot to ask about the mileage for this longer route, but really it didn't matter. I knew he was bored with the freeway route on Interstate 10 that he/we had traveled so many times since November 2005.

Karen was in an uncharacteristically grumpy mood all day. She said no one came in to change her for over an hour in the morning. I didn't understand why she hadn't used her call button more, but suspected she may have fallen asleep after she first tried to summon someone. I wished she had the strength, confidence, concentration, or some other trait, to get out of bed and get cleaned up on her own. I also reflected that perhaps the staff had told her not to do so, fearing she might fall.

I was sure Karen was anxious about all the unknowns, too, such as who would be able to take care of her and where she was going to live, when and if she was going to be reactivated and the big question, which was how much longer until she had a transplant.

Karen went to physical therapy and it was obvious she was getting stronger. In fact she gloated, "They tease me because I go to therapy without being reminded to go." It was a dramatic change from a month earlier when Karen was content to stay in bed!

I left her at the end of the afternoon to go back to the Transplant House to wait for Paul. Very soon after he arrived, we went out to get something to eat. We took Karen's car, and I drove to the restaurant. When we came out, I headed for the driver's seat but Paul insisted on driving. We had decided to go see Karen for a short visit, because I knew she always perked up when she saw him. It was going to be a surprise, though, as I didn't know if Paul was going to feel like visiting after his long day in the car.

Leaving the parking lot, Paul pulled into a left turn lane. At the last minute he turned into the next lane over to the right, which was also a left turn lane. A man in a BMW was accelerating into the same spot, I suppose in a hurry to catch the green light. He swerved to try to avoid us, but the 2 cars sideswiped each other.

We didn't go to see Karen.

If there were reasons for the accident, I would suggest they were that Paul was exhausted, he wasn't accustomed to driving the lumbering bigger car, and we were all stressed out. Anyway, back at the Transplant House, Paul took a quick shower and collapsed into one of the twin beds in the room and was out like a light. I had rearranged the furniture in my Room 6 and had pushed the twin beds together. At least it looked like a King size bed, and for the first time in a long time, I could reach out and touch him.

The next day Paul cleaned up the scrapes on Karen's car, glued the headlight back in, and after lunch, told his sister what happened. She took it remarkably well, saying, "With everything that has been going on and with all you and Jean have been doing for me, I'm not too worried about a few scrapes on a seven-year-old car." She added, "I'll have you to thank when my car insurance rates go up next time!" It was a flash of teasing humor I didn't often see. It was also nice to hear her acknowledgement that she thought we had been doing a lot for her.

By the time Karen and Paul called the insurance company about the incident, the other driver, (a doctor), had already called it in. The Claims person said Paul would be hearing from an adjuster.

Paul talked to Ted Dailey at the Transplant House. We assured him that we would take care of Karen or see that others in the family would be there as caregivers when needed. Paul left messages for Jack Kelly at Mayo. Karen and I talked to Dr. Cho who also talked to Jack Kelly. The outcome of all those various conversations was good news. We learned that Ted had shared with Jack his observation of how mobile Karen had been when he met her on April 4th. Ted and Jack discussed how common it had become (in their experience) for a transplant patient to be temporarily deactivated and reactivated prior to surgery. They decided together it would be okay for Karen to move to the Transplant House with me when she was discharged from the rehab center. Housing there was going to be much easier than having to rent an apartment, rent furniture, etc., or to have to commute back and forth from Green Valley to Phoenix.

Paul had come up with a plan for Karen that could possibly entice someone to come and be her caregiver. He told her that perhaps she could offer a salary and/or a bonus at the end of some number of weeks. Karen immediately made some objections about how expensive that would be. Paul pointed out that it was her life and her future they were discussing, and that she was very fortunate to have sufficient financial resources at her disposal to consider such care, if it came to that. Karen agreed to the approach, and called both her cousin Julie and Lea and told them her offer.

Paul also called his cousin Julie. He was trying to keep all options for Karen's care open. When he spoke to Julie she said she was going to come and take care of Karen! She said that she would just need a couple weeks to get someone to take care of her cats and to talk to her boss about leaving her job, at a company where she had recently been re-hired. Julie called Karen after that, and the two women talked for a long time.

Lea also called Paul, as he had left a message for her on the previous Saturday or Sunday. She kept saying things like, "It's a lot to take in" and "I'd have to leave my life here" and talked about her new job there in Mississippi. I was pretty sure she was going to say no. But Paul let me know that Lea told Karen she had gotten it worked out with her boss to come for 7-8 weeks. As Paul said, "That's something." Maybe if each person could take a few weeks, like Penny did, like we were doing . . .

On Wednesday April 12th we heard from Jack Kelly that Karen was scheduled to have a paracentesis the next day, as well as some appointments on Friday with Jack at 12:50 p.m., and with Dr. Brown at 1:00 p.m.

Thursday was a very long, hot, and ultimately disappointing day. I left the Transplant House at 7:40 a.m. and grabbed a breakfast burrito at a fast food restaurant on the way. I picked Karen up a little after 8:00 and took her out to the Mayo Clinic on Shea Boulevard for her "fasting blood draw" at 8:50. Then we checked in with Radiology and she ate an apple (her breakfast). The staff took her for her paracentesis at 9:50 and she was done about an hour later. I had become accustomed to waiting for long periods of time in waiting rooms at Mayo, and prepared for those times by bringing a newspaper or magazine.

There was a big mix-up about her getting an albumin infusion. There were no orders in the computer; the doctor that did the paracentesis couldn't be found; the folks in Radiology reviewed Karen's computer file and saw she had gotten albumin in March but had not received any in February or January. No one (including me) thought to call Jack Kelly. So we left.

We were too late to get Karen back to her room in time for lunch. She said she was craving a taco, so we went to a nearby restaurant. I sent a text-message to Paul and he joined us there. I finally dropped Karen back to her room so she could take a nap at about 1:45 p.m. Just as I was dreaming of a nap myself; Karen called me on my cell phone. Jack Kelly had called her wanting to know where she was and why she had not gotten the albumin that she was supposed to get. So, off we went again to the Shea Boulevard facility. It took a long time for the albumin to go into Karen's vein. Finally, I dropped a very tired Karen in her room, where, thankfully, her dinner tray was waiting. It was 5 p.m. I began thinking that perhaps because Karen's liver disease had gotten so much worse, maybe the albumin was more important.[19]

We were told 5 liters of fluid had been removed during the paracentesis on that day, April 13th. I did some math and figured out 4 liters weighs 9.6 pounds, 1 liter weighs 2.4 pounds, and 5 liters weighs 12 pounds! As I had suspected before, it must have felt like unstrapping a heavy weight from her abdomen every time Karen had the procedure done. That day we were told if 3 liters or more came off in any paracentesis in the future, there were standing orders for Karen to get the albumin infusion.

After Paul and I watched a little TV, Paul called Julie to offer to drive from New Mexico over to her home in California to pick her up, and then drive her back to Scottsdale, knowing she would be able to use Karen's car while there. Julie said she was very touched by Paul's offer, but said she had found a one-way rental car for $76. That didn't sound too bad.

Then the conversation shifted. While I couldn't hear her voice, from Paul's responses, I could tell she started to talk about not wanting to give up her cats or her job. It was only a day later but she was having second thoughts. Julie said her boss told her if she left she would not be eligible to be re-hired again for two years. Her boss said if she stayed, she would be promoted to assistant director by the end of that year. In the end, Julie said she wasn't coming.

Paul handled it really well. The way they left it was Julie would continue to explore options for the cats, and clarify what her options for a leave of absence from work really were. Paul specifically asked Julie not to call Karen that evening because Karen was exhausted from her procedures and from the long and trying day.

My heart sank. Once again, it looked to me like it was going to be the two of us for the duration. I knew Paul and I couldn't abandon Karen, and that Paul couldn't stay there with me (or with us) the whole time because he had various duties with respect to running his company, not to mention the care of our own cats. My hopes were up, my hopes were dashed.

Chapter 15

Advocate (noun), Advocate (verb)

On Friday, April 14, 2006, Karen, Paul and I went to Mayo. Karen had gotten a haircut in the beauty shop at the nursing home the day before, and had put gel in her hair for the appointment. She had chosen a mint-green over shirt and had applied a little makeup. She walked in with her walker, and that impressed Jack Kelly. He said, "Look at you, you're a new woman, all coiffed." Then Jack suggested, "When Dr. Brown comes into the room, why don't you stand and shake his hand?" And Karen did. It was a great moment.

Dr. Brown said he had reviewed the hematology report, as well as the results of the paracentesis the day before. Dr. Brown confirmed the conclusions I had drawn the previous week when Karen and I had met the hematology specialist. Karen's abnormalities in blood clotting which were due to End Stage Liver Disease *would be resolved with a transplant.* The next good news came when the doctor said he was impressed with Karen's progress walking and getting her strength back. He said she was very lucky to have family supporting her. Even though Paul and I were continuing to work on getting additional caregivers for the future, we had effectively played our roles as committed caregivers at the Transplant House and at Karen's various doctor appointments.

It was nice to hear this doctor summarize the positive progress on all the important issues with respect to Karen's situation. However, he cautioned us that "rehab" as defined at a skilled nursing facility is described only as "what insurance will cover". We clearly got the message that Karen had to keep up with her walking and strength-building exercises.

Dr. Brown said it was his job to be an advocate for Karen at the Transplant Committee meeting the next week. He said he hoped to get Karen reactivated on the transplant list. Paul heard that and knew that it was one thing to have an assigned role of being an advocate and quite another actually to advocate in the committee meeting. So Paul asked pointedly, "*Will you* advocate for her?" Dr. Brown said, "Yes, I will."

After the doctor left the room, Jack reviewed Karen's file (on the computer) and said Karen's MELD score was twenty-four, (up from twenty-two) and it could go higher due to the tumor in her liver. Jack said the score right then was based, in part, on two of three blood factors, bilyrubin and clotting, which were abnormal, but not on the third factor, creatinine, which for the time being was okay. Elevated creatinine, I had learned, made a MELD score go up because it indicates problems with kidney functioning. Although it can be done, a transplant team in general does not want a patient to need both a new liver *and* a new kidney.

There was also a discussion about whether Karen's filter was a removable one, and Jack said he would follow up on that. It was noted that if it were not removable, Karen would need to be followed post-transplant with anti-coagulation drugs, such as Coumadin. This upset Karen as it had done in the appointment with Dr. Gossett, but Paul and I later reassured her that weekly or monthly blood draws and fiddling with the dosage of that particular drug would all be very do-able.

During that day's doctor visit it finally seemed the issues about Karen's deactivated status were being addressed. A transplant would solve the "blood clot business," even if she would have to take anti-coagulation drugs for the rest of her life. I had been living at the Transplant House for weeks and Paul had driven to Phoenix four times since the first of March; clearly we were regarded as Karen's caregivers. Karen was up and walking; her determination was obvious to the people at the nursing home, to Jack Kelly, to Dr. Brown, and to us. Dr. Brown had asserted he would be an advocate for Karen when the Transplant Committee met the following week. It was remarkable.

After the appointment was finished, Paul guided Karen with her walker down to the Mayo Hospital cafeteria and told her she might be hearing from their cousin soon. He gave her the news that Julie likely would not be able to give up her new job or to leave her cats to come to Arizona for a period of time. Karen was disappointed, to say the least. It was so typical to have bad news about the caregiver situation in the same day as getting optimistic news about the doctor being her advocate at the next transplant committee meeting.

We took Karen back to her room at the nursing home. Paul and I discussed whether we would take a trip down to Karen's house in Green Valley, but decided not to do that. Too much driving. Instead, we told Karen she would not see us at all the next day. I needed a break. It had been four weeks since I had stayed for the first time at the Transplant House. Everything that was happening was so intense. Even though I didn't have constant care of Karen, she was on my mind all the time, every day.

On Saturday Paul and I went to an IKEA store in Tempe, Arizona. We walked around for almost three hours. We saw items we thought we might want to purchase at some time in the future, perhaps to replace a couch. Even though we talked about Karen and her situation throughout the day, it was nice to have a day off. I knew that the unknown portion of Karen's situation, never knowing when or if she would get transplant surgery, was the most difficult challenge.

The day after our shopping trip, Paul and I went to breakfast at the Mayo Hospital Cafeteria. It has good food and good prices. Then we went to a bookstore. Karen called on my cell phone and told me Lea's friend Marcia had agreed to come from Mississippi and take care of her. Lea had given a lot of thought to her mother's predicament, and thought of her friend, who was available to travel to Arizona. Lea wanted to help solve the problem of a caregiver and Marcia wanted to take care of Karen. In addition, she liked the idea of having an income for a number of weeks.

Marcia had asked Karen if she'd be able to leave her at least for a few hours at a time. While I had been doing that in the evenings while living at the Transplant House, I wasn't sure how easy it would be for Marcia to get away after Karen was released from the nursing home. Karen told us confidently she had assured Marcia she would be able to leave and go visit a friend, go to the movies, etc. I took it as a good sign that Karen could envision herself on her own for periods of time. I was optimistic about Marcia's arrival. For the first time in a long time I felt the worry about Karen's situation subtly shifting to a more manageable level.

In the afternoon we took Karen to a store to buy a pair of sandals. Karen had only one pair of shoes with her (and a pair of slippers) so we were pretty sure the sandals would be a big improvement to help her be steady on her feet. They had good straps and Karen said they were comfortable as soon as she put them on. She had hammertoes and bunions on her feet, so finding good, comfortable shoes was difficult.

Paul left for home on the morning of Monday, April 17. The night before he had listened to a number of voice messages on our phone at home. He said one call had been some advice, but he didn't want to say who had called. He knew it would upset me so he said he'd tell me about it the next morning. That was an excellent decision; when I heard the message I was livid. It seems someone felt compelled to tell Paul that it was *his* responsibility to take care of his sister. What had we been doing? We had been heavily involved in Karen and Dave's lives over the previous couple of years, and that involvement was continuing. How easy it was to second-guess us with respect to the care of Karen. And to leave it on the message machine instead of saying it directly to Paul. I eventually got over it but I couldn't believe we were dealing with that along with everything else. No one was behaving normally, that was for sure.

Paul coached Karen before he left for home. He reminded her to concentrate on increasing her strength and to work on being able to step up a couple of stairs, up on a curb, and up on an examining table. The next day Karen asked one of the physical therapists to work with her on those things. She was *so focused* on getting and staying strong, and I think she wanted to please Paul.

Karen said she talked to Marcia in Mississippi. I had suggested that the two of them should decide on some start and end dates so that we could get an airline ticket for a good fare, and so Marcia would know exactly what the timeframe was going to be for her stay. Marcia agreed to come out for 8 weeks. I also suggested that Karen could begin to plan what to do for a companion, and who that might be, after Marcia's time was up. I still had in the back of my mind the six-month estimate until transplant that had been given to us by the social worker.

In the evening I signed onto the Internet and found a round-trip airline ticket for a good price. When I called and told Karen the cost she said, "Use my credit card and go ahead and book it as soon as you can."

That night at the Transplant House the couple from Pinetop made spaghetti for everyone. There were 10 people in the dining room, including the newest arrival, a man who had received a pancreas transplant, staying there with his friend and caregiver. The man from Pinetop had received his transplant on March 25, and was scheduled to go home on April 20. As Ted Dailey, Transplant House Director said, he was "the poster boy" for liver transplant surgery. He and his wife had cooked a celebratory dinner; it was really nice.

Early the next morning I spent a couple of hours booking the round trip airplane tickets on the computer at the Arizona Transplant House. Marcia was scheduled to fly to Phoenix on May 2 and home to Mississippi on June 27. I had offered to stick around for a while, helping Karen train Marcia on the various aspects of her condition, her medications, her exercise requirements, etc. The time Marcia would spend in Arizona would take care of 8 weeks into the future, a portion of the time that had been on my mind since attending the Liver Transplant Support Group meeting earlier that month.

While I was working on getting the airline ticket booked, Karen had a great session with Dr. Cho at the nursing home. He told her she would be able to be discharged in two days, on Thursday, April 20, 2006. He commended her on her progress since her arrival on March 8th, and wished her well. He ordered her a walker. He said her prescriptions would be ready for her when she checked out on Thursday.

In the afternoon a box of mail arrived from Norma, who had shipped it from Green Valley before she started a 6-week vacation. Karen was feeling a little under-the-weather with a queasy stomach. She ate some crackers, drank some room-temperature ginger ale, and I arranged for some chicken broth and rice to be sent to her room for supper. It had been one of my many roles since I moved to Scottsdale in March; being Karen's legs.

I also was her voice, especially when it was too difficult for her to articulate her needs and her wishes. I had gotten so I could read her pretty well, and tried to imagine what I would want if I were in her place. I had learned to ask her a lot of questions, like "would you like me to . . .", always aware that I didn't want to overstep my bounds and make her more upset about the things she wasn't able, or perhaps willing, to do on her own. It was exhausting for both of us, and sometimes rewarding for me, all at the same time.

There had been a crisis of one sort or another nearly every day. I routinely had tried really hard not to feel overwhelmed. Each day I had to try to put the latest crisis out of my mind so I could get ready for the next day and prepare to meet whatever happened with a fresh outlook. Like Penny before me, I was beginning to feel the relief that would come when Marcia arrived and took over.

On Wednesday I brought Karen's checkbook and briefcase to her. She had gone through all the mail that had arrived the day before. She'd read her credit card bill, but couldn't remember authorizing one charge for a large amount that was described as "co-pay for inpatient Skilled Nursing Care" on the day she was discharged from the Tucson facility. She called me on the cell phone while I was in the middle of making my lunch at the Transplant House. Rather than blurt out all her business in one of the common areas, I suggested we could talk about it more when I arrived at her room in about an hour. I should have confirmed it *was* a legitimate charge; I was there the day she signed for it before she checked out of the nursing home in Tucson, the day we moved her to Scottsdale.

Since she still could not recognize the charge amount, Karen called the credit card company, said the amount was in dispute, and cancelled the card! I knew that action would make more of a project later, but it was done, so I didn't say anything. On the other hand, it was some independent action and responsible thinking I hadn't seen in her in a long while. She had written out all her other checks for the bills that came in the package, a daunting exercise for someone who is well. It was one she hadn't done since December, four months earlier.

There were a lot of smiling faces at the Transplant House. Two couples, both the people from Douglas and the folks from Pinetop were scheduled to go home the next day. The man from Pinetop told Paul and me that his liver transplant was estimated to be worth $750,000 and, since he was a Disabled Vietnam Era Veteran, so far he hadn't paid a dime. Wow.

I spent a lot of time in the afternoon packing Karen's things and making numerous trips from her room at the rehab center to the parking lot to load the car. It was a good thing it had such a huge trunk and large back seat! I realized Karen had been in one rehab center or another for nearly 12 weeks, since the day I held her hand and said we would find a place for her to stay. Anyway, she had accumulated a lot of stuff! That evening I packed my things, as I was going to be moving out of little Room 6. I had rearranged the twin beds, moving the furniture back the way it was when I had moved in.

The plan was to go to Karen's house in Green Valley for a couple of days, and then go back together to The Arizona Transplant House to a larger room. Then we would wait for Marcia's arrival on May 2, wait to hear from the Mayo doctors if Karen had been reactivated, and finally wait for a call saying a liver was available. Karen and I were both moving on to a new phase, leaving behind the routines that had been our existence since the early part of March.

Chapter 16

A Big Day

The date was April 20, 2006, a Thursday, and I was awake before the alarm went off at 6:30. I had promised Karen the day before that I would be at her room between 8:15 and 8:30 a.m. I sent her a text-message saying I was bringing her a strawberry milkshake. I finished loading up the back seat of the car with my suitcases and bags. I left my key and a note for Ted and took a picture (with my cell phone) of the little room that had been my home for all those weeks. I sent a text-message to Paul that I was all packed. I made the milkshakes and was out the door at 8:15 a.m., thinking it was going to be a big day for Karen.

On the way in the car my cell phone rang, but it was in my purse in the back seat, so I couldn't get to it. When I parked the car and looked at the "missed calls" log, it showed "no number" so I didn't call back.

As I was approaching Karen's room, I saw her walking toward the nurse's station. She was checking on her prescriptions and her discharge paperwork. They were still working on them. So we went to her room to enjoy the milkshakes, all the more because Karen had not received a breakfast tray.

It flitted through my mind that we should call Jack at Mayo, because the transplant committee had met the day before.

A few minutes later, Karen's cell phone rang, and I heard her say "Hi Paul" while glancing at me. Karen said, "Oh, I am?" I just knew she had been re-activated. It was true. Paul explained that Jack had called Karen, then me, then Paul, to give us the news. So *that* was my missed call!

Paul reminded both of us to keep our cell phones charged and handy at all times. Paul sent me a text-message that read, "Jack said the entire team was very impressed with the effort Karen has put in to get back on the active list." What a wonderful start to the day! I did a little dance in Karen's room. She said she'd be dancing, too, if she thought she could be sure she wouldn't lose her balance.

Around 9:30 Karen signed herself out, received nine prescriptions, and said her goodbyes. She'd been told her walker had been ordered and would be delivered to the Arizona Transplant House the following week. She also was told insurance would cover some therapy sessions there and a therapist would be calling her to schedule them. We put another bag of clothing and other assorted items on the wheelchair Karen had been using. She pushed it to the front door and parked it there. Then she walked (without a walker) with me to the car.

We were on the road heading south by 9:50 a.m. Around 11:00 a.m. Karen's cell phone rang and it was Jack calling from Mayo. He said Karen needed to have a CT scan for her chest, and asked us to turn around and come back. His request really threw Karen. She had been looking forward to spending two nights and parts of three days at her house. She'd made up an impossibly long list of things to do. After Karen explained all that, Jack said he would make a few inquiries and call Karen back.

When Jack called again he said he had set up the CT scan for the next day, Friday. He said, "We want you within two hours of Mayo." We found that comment to be curious because Karen had told him that morning we were going to Green Valley and returning to the Arizona Transplant House on Saturday, when our room would be ready.

Meanwhile, as Karen was talking in the car, I decided to pull off the highway and stop at a station to get some gasoline. Karen handed me a credit card. It turned out to be the credit card she had cancelled, but she hadn't remembered doing that. I didn't know which card she had handed me, and didn't think to ask which one it was. I walked into the building requesting that a manager approve the transaction twice before Karen realized she could give me a different card to use. It was one of those frustrating, time-consuming things that I had learned to deal with and promptly put behind me.

I called Paul and told him about Jack's call, and called the Arizona Transplant House to see if we could have our room on the next day, on Friday, one day earlier than previously planned. "Yes," Donna told us, "the room will be ready tomorrow." Then I talked Karen into sharing a sandwich; I was hungry. We bought soft drinks and got back into the car again.

As we approached Green Valley at about 1:15 p.m., Karen suggested that we drop her prescriptions off at the pharmacy. She walked into the building, greeted the pharmacist for the first time in a long time, and walked back out to the car. Then I drove to the house. We had decided not to unpack everything. Karen had made *another* list in the car, in addition to the lists she had made earlier in the week. So we were about to combine lists and get started on the Things to Do. My first priority, though, was to make a quick trip to a bathroom.

As I walked through Karen's house, her cell phone rang again. She had just walked into her kitchen for the first time in months. With a muttered, "Oh, God Bless," she answered the phone. When I heard her formal response, "Yes, this is she" and a series of "no" and "yes" answers, I left her to it and shut the door to the bathroom. A few minutes later I emerged and glanced at Karen. She had an odd look on her face.

"We have to go back to Phoenix," she said.

"Now what?" I asked, with more than a little irritation in my voice.

"That was Mayo," she said calmly. "They have a liver. They said they'll be doing the donor's surgery at 5:00 p.m. and we should hurry back. They said we shouldn't kill ourselves getting there." And she gave a little laugh.

I shrieked! Even though I'd been thinking since the appointment with the hematology specialist that Karen would be reactivated and then get her liver soon, I never thought it would be *that* day! She had just been reactivated the day before and released from the extended care facility that morning! It was too much to absorb!

I called Paul and told him Mayo had a liver.

"No shit?" he shouted. Here was the answer to all our prayers and hopes. It was actually happening!

Karen and I packed up three lighter-weight pairs of slacks, some short-sleeve blouses, 2 pairs of shoes, some bath towels and two pillows. As I was throwing all that into the car, Karen called the pharmacy and cancelled her prescriptions. She also called her neighbor and asked her to take care of something there at her house. Karen had been instructed not to eat or drink. I grabbed a can of soda out of her refrigerator and, at 2:02 p.m., less than an hour after arriving in Green Valley . . . and like the Willy Nelson song, we were "On The Road Again."

In the car Karen had a wonderful time calling people and telling them her stories of the day, being reactivated, driving home, getting The Call. It was unreal, hard to grasp, and totally amazing all at the same time. Every few minutes in the car I would chuckle again at Paul's shouted reaction. Karen and I made up other responses I could have said to him like, "Just kidding" or "We were practicing for the time when the *real* call comes." We were silly and happy and so excited.

Karen called Norma with the news. Norma called back a few minutes later saying she wanted to be sure it wasn't a dream. Paul called on Karen's cell phone a little after 4 p.m. to caution us about Phoenix rush-hour traffic. She handed me the phone briefly so he could remind me to be really careful about my driving. I assured him that I was very focused and aware. I told him I was in some kind of alert, intent driving zone—every nerve was firing because it was such a critical run in the car—for the second time that day.

Some time during the ride I told Karen about the dream I'd had back at the end of January. I told her the vivid details, including her walking toward me, steady on her feet, slimmed down from the abdominal fluid, smiling, walking next to a white building on a large grassy yard, and that she was well. I told her I didn't recognize the setting at the time but as soon as I moved into the Arizona Transplant House, there it was: The grassy area was the back yard; the white building was the stucco garage. Karen just grinned as I told her. I knew it would be a good image for her to hold as she went into surgery.

Karen spent some time in the car going through more mail. She seemed serene. I was amazed that she could focus. It was wonderful, because reading her mail did pass some time and I was able to concentrate completely on my driving. Karen called Jack again, and received some additional admitting instructions.

I had to make a quick restroom stop on Interstate-10, just south of the exit for Route 587. That break took fewer than six minutes (I timed myself) because I *ran* in and out. I was in a hurry both because of the excitement and because I needed the exercise, to be sure I was wide-awake and alert.

During the previous couple of weeks Paul had encouraged Karen to write some things down in case she didn't get a liver or in case she didn't make it through a surgery. As her brother and the one most likely to be involved with executing her wishes, he wanted to know what to do about certain things. He had researched how to do a hand-written will, and Micki had reluctantly written a few things down.

On Route 202 and Route 101, we saw a lot of traffic heading south away from Phoenix. Heading north, we only had to slow down for traffic once when we approached the Scottsdale Road exit, only four miles from our destination. I was glad we had stopped and filled the gas tank that morning. As we pulled into the Mayo parking lot I realized I did not want to drop Karen off near the front door by herself. I asked her if she wanted to take her hand-written will, which we had discussed in the car, with her into the hospital.

"No. Leave it. I think I'm going to be fine."

I thought it would be good for Karen to walk one more time. So I parked and asked Karen, "Is this going to be okay?" When she hesitated, I reminded her of all the times she had been told she needed to be able to walk on her own to be eligible for transplant surgery. She nodded. I could see the determination on her face.

As we opened our doors to get out of the car, we became aware of the rotor-blade-thumping and wind of a helicopter landing there at Mayo. One of us exclaimed, "Maybe that's the liver arriving!" It was close to 5 p.m., and Karen had been told the donor's surgery was going to be done at about that time, so it was actually too early. But it was a strange moment. I'm sure Karen was thinking what I was thinking. There was grief and sadness in another family on the same day we were feeling so elated.

As Karen and I walked into the front doors, I realized I was so proud of her. She walked into Mayo Hospital for her transplant, on my arm, at her own pace, no walker. It was a great beginning. But she was thirsty and tired, so I began to look for a wheelchair. By 5:15 p.m. she was being wheeled to a room.

Then the waiting began. Someone was helping Karen get into a gown just as Dr. Brown arrived. I could tell he was pretty excited, too. Just as a nurse had done minutes before, he cautioned Karen that the liver might not be acceptable. He also discussed the risks of surgery, as well as the additional risks of possible rejection and/or possible complications of transplant surgery. Since Karen had been through so many hospital visits and surgeries in her lifetime, she was very well aware of all the risks. She said, "Yes, I know" and "Yes, I understand" throughout the discussion. The doctor asked if either of us had any additional questions.

"While I'm under, I was wondering, could someone do a facelift?" Karen said, with a straight face. Then she grinned. After a lot of laughter, Dr. Brown said, simply, "no."

"No one ever asked *that* question before!" he allowed.

He explained that the donor's heart was being prepared for another patient, so Karen's surgery would follow. The new estimated time for her operation was going to be delayed, from 10 p.m. until 1 a.m.

"It doesn't matter; we'll be here," I quipped.

When Karen and I were alone again, each of us kept commenting on how incredible the turn of events was. It was what everyone was hoping for and waiting for, but it was still difficult to grasp once the time had arrived.

Karen was wheeled away for x-rays, taken into the shower, and repeatedly poked for what seemed like fifty tubes of blood. At 7 p.m. we settled down to watch some of our favorite TV shows: Survivor Panama/Exile Island, CSI (the original, set in Las Vegas), and Without a Trace (thank you, CBS). At 10 p.m. we turned to a movie channel and watched "Ace Ventura, Pet Detective," a Jim Carrey movie.

Shortly after midnight Paul sent me a text-message to say he had arrived at the Arizona Transplant House, quite a fast drive for him from Alamogordo to Scottsdale. He probably found himself in that focused driving zone too, in spite of the fact he had just made the same drive, in the other direction, three days earlier. Since it felt like 1 a.m. to him, I encouraged him to catch some sleep, and said I could send a text-message if I needed him.

Chapter 17

Transplant

At 12:30 a.m. two nurses came in with a wheelchair and one of them said, "Are you ready?" Karen moved toward the edge of the bed and was on her feet in no time. I quickly gathered up my things and followed. When we reached a set of doors, one of the nurses said, "Here's where you can say goodbye."

"Okay sweetie, good luck, and I'll see you when you wake up," I said. The nurses said if it turned out that they were able to come and get me for another quick visit, it would be in the next twenty to forty minutes. So I made myself comfortable in a waiting area near those doors.

No one came.

About an hour later someone else came by and said the cafeteria was open so I went down and ate again. Since I knew I wouldn't be getting much sleep, I decided I must be hungry. There's something about lack of sleep that made me want to compensate with food and drink. At about 2:20 a.m. an Operating Room nurse came out to say Karen's surgery began at 2:16 a.m. She asked me if I was going to stay all night, and when I said yes, suggested that I try to get some sleep. She took me to a room near the Second Floor Intensive Care Unit where specialized chairs folded out to be narrow and surprisingly comfortable beds. The room was dark and others were already asleep. The nurse also gave me two warmed flannel sheets. They were wonderful. When I first lay down, I didn't think I'd be able to sleep. But with the warm sheets to relax me, I finally drifted off.

At 4:35 a.m. the same nurse from the OR came by to tell me Karen's liver had been removed and that the surgeon was starting to sew the new liver in. Since I had been asleep and didn't know what a normal schedule was, I thought things were moving along very well. I stayed on the chair-bed until 5 a.m. When I realized I wouldn't be able to sleep again, I moved out to another waiting area on the Second Floor, near the elevators. With a flannel sheet still around my shoulders, I wrote notes about that incredible Thursday. As the day grew brighter and the sun came up, I had an overwhelming sense that getting the new liver was a great new beginning for Karen.

At 6:07 a.m. on April 21, 2006, the OR nurse (a person whose name I never learned) came looking for me and found me in my new location. She said the two surgeons were preparing to close. She said Karen had lost a lot of blood during surgery, but was doing okay. She said one or both of the doctors would be out to see me shortly, and asked me to stay where I was near the elevators. For the next fifty-three minutes I barely moved; I didn't want to miss that conversation.

At 7 a.m. Dr. Morton came out and told me Karen received the right lobe and part of the left lobe of a teenager donor's liver. He said another surgeon flew into Arizona and obtained the other portion of the liver for a baby in California. I thought, "Two lives saved by this one organ!" Dr. Morton explained Karen had been chosen to receive the liver because of her size and her blood group. He said it took a long time to remove Karen's liver because of adhesions all along her scar from the splenectomy she had back in 1986. He said when he had to move her intestines in order to get at her liver, it was as if the intestines and her skin were glued together, and when he had to pull them apart, it caused a scrape which in turn caused bleeding, or oozing. When I asked how much blood she had lost, he said he didn't know. He said there was about a ten percent chance he would have to take her back into surgery in the first twenty-four hours to clean up the oozing blood in her abdomen. He said once she got to the Intensive Care Unit (ICU) and got warmed up, the bleeding would probably stop on its own.

He said Karen was still in the Operating Room, that she was still intubated, and that she would be going to ICU soon. He said the sewing in of the new liver was "actually pretty mechanical" and went as was to be expected. He said I should go and get some rest and visit

Karen after lunch in the ICU. I thanked Dr. Morton "for her and for the whole family." He said, "You're very welcome."

We talked about what an amazing journey it had been and he said he was reminded of that notion with each patient. He commented that his surgeries were wondrous for him every time. He said another doctor would be taking over the rotation starting that day (Friday) and would be the surgeon looking in on Karen in ICU. Dr. Morton said he'd be looking in, too, more to say hello than for a surgical reason.

After Dr. Morton left me I took the elevator down and walked out to the front of the hospital, where I could see the sun climbing in the eastern sky, the same view I'd had outside the elevators on the second floor. I sent a text-message to Paul, and one by one, called Penny, Norma and Grace on the phone. Each woman was overjoyed to hear Karen's surgery had gone well. Paul sent a text-message back to me and said he was on his way to the hospital. But I quickly responded, asking him not to come, saying instead that I would meet him at the Transplant House. When I got there, Paul was sitting at the dining room table. We talked about the previous twenty-four hours. I was exhausted but not sleepy. Finally I took a shower and tried to sleep. Late in the morning after resting for a while, Paul and I went out for something to eat.

We visited Karen for a short while in Room 17 in the Intensive Care Unit, putting on paper gowns, gloves and masks. She was still very groggy, barely able to stay awake. She had so many tubes, two down her nose and several in each hand and arm. I think I counted 19 things attached to her! Right after surgery most patients are really scared. So much has happened to their bodies, and they are in a lot of pain. It is ***nothing*** like what you see on TV.

Even though the patient receives pain medication, there is another factor, a *will to live*, that must be in the patient's mind and spirit to get through a really difficult few days. This "will to live" surely must be a big part of what the selection committee looks for in patients who are selected for transplants. I believe Karen demonstrated her will to live by working hard at walking again while in Scottsdale.

Paul and I were immediately impressed with the skills of Karen's first ICU nurse, a woman named Gail. She said she'd been working in the transplant ICU area for ten years. We were encouraged that she really knew what to watch for and, more importantly, *what to do* for her patient. It was not an intensive care unit where a nurse had several patients in her care. The needs of the patient were so extreme and the necessary skills of the nurse on duty were so extraordinary that Karen was the nurse's only patient. The patient didn't need a family member to be her advocate and protector; the nurse **was** her professional advocate. Each ICU nurse worked a 12-hour shift, so each one provided extensive, intensive care for a long period of time in the patient's recovery. All Karen's nurses were extremely skilled; we know Mayo attracts and retains top-notch personnel.

Paul and I were very concerned about a note on the white board in Karen's room. It said "tumor in stomach removed during transplant." We asked Gail what that meant. She said we would have to talk to a doctor. We had learned to put information like that on the back burner; we would deal with it later.

We didn't stay long and Gail said we were wise to go. She said the most important thing for Karen right then was to rest and recover. She said she didn't need the germs or the distraction of having us in her room, trying to talk or trying to stay awake for us. Gail also reaffirmed our thoughts that our important job would follow that of the nurses, so we didn't need to be there then. In addition, Karen wouldn't remember much about her stay in the intensive care unit.

That evening I talked to Lea. She cried tears of relief that her mom had gotten her transplant and that she wasn't going to lose another parent, at least not yet. She said it truly felt like an incredible new beginning, and thanked me for being there for her mother.

The first full day after surgery, Saturday, April 22, 2006, was a blur. Paul and I visited Karen, donning gowns and gloves for the second time. "One size fits none" is what someone in the ICU called the gowns when he helped us with them. Karen's color was good (that was what I noticed). She was having trouble talking with the tubes down her throat, and said she was in a lot of pain. Her nurse, Darlene, said that day would be her roughest day. As Paul related to someone after our visit, Karen had a sparkle in her eyes that hadn't been there for a long time. She was resolute. She would get through it.

When one of the intravenous (IV) needles was removed from Karen's right wrist, a nerve was damaged. She held a warm pack on the inside of her wrist during one of our visits. The doctors were concerned about some red spots on Karen's right thumb, but I assured them she had those before. Karen clarified, rasping, "I've had those spots for twenty-five years".

Karen's ICU nurse from the first day, Gail, had advised us to visit early on Saturday so we would have a better chance of seeing the doctors. When we arrived at the ICU her doctor was not in, but Karen was up walking! She was going from her bedside to the desk at the nurse's station, perhaps a distance of eighteen feet, and back. It was an amazing feat just twenty-five hours after her surgery had ended. The look I saw on Karen's face was a mixture of pain and grim determination. The process took three people to help her *and* manage all the equipment. Karen later spent several hours sitting up in the chair next to her bed. We were told the pathology report on the tumor would be back on Monday.

Melinda, mother of Karen's grandchildren, called me on Saturday afternoon. Lea had called her so Caroline, Ron and she would have news of Karen's transplant. Randy called on Karen's cell phone at his usual weekly time. Since I had Karen's phone with me, I was able to tell him the big news and some of the amazing details of Karen's day on Thursday. Like the rest of us, he said he was having a hard time absorbing it all. He kept repeating how glad he was, and he sent his love.

Sunday, April 23, 2006 was the second day after surgery. It began for Paul and me very early with a phone call from Karen's ICU nurse of the day, Krista. She quickly cautioned us not to be concerned that she was calling and told us Karen was unreasonably concerned about some of the things she was hearing. Krista assured me again everything was okay.

"For some reason, Karen heard me say that her urine output was down," Krista continued. "As Karen became really focused on that statistic, she insisted I notify her family." Krista suggested we could reassure Karen when we visited, and say she was getting the fluids she needed intravenously, her output was fine, and everything was on track as it was supposed to be.

So Paul and I showered and got going, arriving at the hospital within an hour. We once again put on gowns and gloves, and soothed Karen's worries. Karen kept repeating, "My counts are down" but when we asked the nurses again, they reassured us that everything was okay. It was a tape that kept playing in her head for some reason. I wondered if all the drugs in her system affected her thoughts and worries.

I noticed that Karen had fewer tubes, but was still uncomfortable with the ones called nasal-gastric, or NG. They were the ones down her throat and taped to her nose. Paul and I left late in the morning to get some food; when I had stood up I felt light-headed. It was not surprising. We all had been through a lot. Once fed, I decided I wanted to go back and see Karen again, so Paul dropped me off at the hospital. Krista told Karen and me that a tray of clear liquids had been ordered. When it arrived, I helped Karen sip juice, clear broth, and ginger ale through a straw.

As she finished each of the items Karen instructed me, "Now put the ones I'm done with at the back of the tray and the ones that are left in the front." She still had some gelatin, iced tea, water, and some of the ginger ale in the front row of the tray. Karen was taking a break from sipping when her nurse came back into the room. She explained what had happened. She had shut down the stomach feeding tube right after Paul and I had left earlier, and had required Karen to wait forty-five minutes before receiving clear liquids by mouth. She said waiting was needed to be certain Karen didn't get nauseated. Hearing all that, I advised Karen to continue but to sip slowly.

Looking at the tray, Krista asked, "How did we do?"

"She had all the soup, all the juice, and half of the ginger ale," I said. Karen nodded in agreement, and watched intently as Krista moved everything around on the tray. Krista checked a few other things in Karen's room, removed her gown and gloves, and went back out to the nurses' station.

"She didn't know our system at all, did she?" Karen asked. I moved everything back, and Karen asked for another sip of ginger ale. Karen's focus on her instructions about how to line things up on her tray was a hilarious example of the behaviors and thought processes of someone on morphine and other drugs. Much later, Karen and I laughed about it.

Paul returned after about ninety minutes.

"I'm not ready for my cell phone yet," Karen announced.

"Good—because you're not getting it!" Paul and I replied in unison.

After Paul's brief visit with Karen, I told both of them I needed to find a bathroom, so Paul and I left. As we walked away from Karen's room, I realized I was totally exhausted! My respect for the ICU nurses grew even more. I understood why it's called <u>intensive</u> care.

On Monday, April 24, 2006, there was still no word on the pathology report. However, another member of the liver transplant team, Dr. Patel, explained that when they had done the Chemo-Embolization to try to shrink the tumor in the liver the previous October, that process had moved the tumor over against the wall of the liver next to the stomach wall. At least that explained why it was being called a tumor in the stomach. Our concern level came down a little; we *had* known all along about that tumor. Dr. Patel also explained that when the surgeon removed Karen's 'old' liver, he also scraped the stomach wall to be sure there was no cancer *in* the stomach. All of this sounded like very good news. We had learned to take each crisis as it came, and if we didn't know what we were dealing with, we didn't borrow trouble prematurely.

That day Karen was given a full liquid diet that included milk, yogurt, ice cream, and tomato soup. She also received word at the end of the afternoon that she would be moved to a regular room that evening. It startled me to realize Karen had spent fewer than seventy-two hours in Intensive Care. Before I left I remembered to give Karen her eyeglasses.

"That makes me feel so much better!" she exclaimed. It was amazing how little things make such a difference on the road to recovery.

Paul happened to run into Jack in a corridor in the Mayo hospital. He said Karen qualified for that particular liver, in part, because of the paracentesis that had been done on April 13, which had gotten her weight down approximately twelve pounds. He also said she became eligible for that liver because she had worked so hard at becoming more ambulatory prior to her discharge from the nursing home on April 20. It was confirmation about our theory about a patient's will to live and ability to fight for a transplant. Of course we knew the resolution of the blood clot business was a huge factor, too. Paul marveled at how many things had come together in just the right way at just the right time to make the surgery possible for his sister.

Karen was moved to a regular hospital room very late in the afternoon on that Monday, April 24th, fewer than four days after her surgery ended on early Friday morning. The next four days were very busy. Karen was encouraged to get up and walk out of her room and around the nurse's station in her ward. She started to eat regular food; her appetite had always been good and it continued to be good that week in the hospital. As soon as the new liver had been transplanted, the need for the prescription laxative ceased. The new liver began working as it should, removing toxins, including ammonia. The side effect of encephalopathy seemed to be gone. Her bathroom visits became normal and routine. (I have often said prayers of thanks that I did not have to spend even one day helping Karen with the frequent diarrhea, which had become such an unpleasant part of her daily life.)

Karen was told her new nurse coordinator for post-transplant care was Jodie Gonzalez, RN. Jodie told Karen that hers was only the third 'split-liver' transplant done at Mayo in Phoenix. She also said Karen was Liver Transplant Patient number 316 since Mayo/Phoenix began doing liver transplants in 1999.

There was a lengthy education process for both of us. We were given a three-ring binder and told to keep all Karen's important papers in it. There was a section for her 'itineraries', which was the word used at Mayo to list scheduled appointments for a patient in the days and weeks to come. There was a section for her medication diary, as there were different dosage and frequency schedules for thirteen medications (initially). Some medicines, such as prednisone, were to be taken on a changing and tapering schedule. Some medicines were to be taken with eight ounces of water; others were to be taken with food. Each day Karen and I would have to check the schedule to make sure we were following all the instructions exactly.

There was a section for her other discharge instructions. There was so much information that Jodie dedicated an entire afternoon discussing these things with Karen and me. Some of those instructions (in no particular order) were:[20]

Karen would be seen about twice a week for four to six weeks after she was discharged from the hospital. Once Karen was released from Mayo and sent home to Green Valley, she would have to have weekly lab/blood tests for a while. Following that and for the rest of the first year she would have to go in to a lab in Green Valley every other week for lab tests. Eventually the frequency would change to monthly lab tests (for the rest of her life). The results would be sent to Mayo; the blood tests would reveal how well the liver was doing and whether there were any signs of rejection.

Karen's caregiver would have to monitor Karen's vital signs, including blood pressure, temperature, and daily weight, as well as keep a record of her medication doses and the time she took them. Immunosuppressive/anti-rejection medication was to be taken one hour after eating OR it was to be taken one hour before eating. All daily statistics needed to be recorded in the 3-ring binder, and the binder was to be taken with us to all Mayo appointments.

We were to report any weight gain of 3 pounds or more overnight.

Blood pressure was to be within a range of (low) 100/60 to (high) 160/90, or Jodie was to be notified immediately.

We were to watch for wound changes, nausea or vomiting, headache, tremors in hands, a fever higher than 102 degrees, diarrhea, a cold or congestion, sweats or chills, shortness of breath, bloody urine or stools or bleeding from any source, skin problems, pain in the chest, persistent cough, leg cramps, or abdominal discomfort, which could be signs of infection and/or rejection.

Since Karen was going to be on immunosuppressive drugs, we were to wash our hands with antibacterial soap often. We were advised Karen should not shake hands with anyone. We were told Karen should stay away from people with upper respiratory illness or other communicable illnesses, especially during the first six months after transplant. Karen was told if she did get sick she should call a doctor within two or three days from then on, and *not* wait a week like other people do when they become sick.

We were told not to share towels, toothbrushes, eating utensils or razors because Karen still has Hepatitis C, and it is a blood borne virus.

We were told to wash all fruits and vegetables. Karen was told not to eat from any salad bars or buffet spreads for the first six months.

Karen was not to handle cleaning products or be in dusty environments. She was to avoid dog kisses and to have someone else pick up doggie poop (or wear a mask and use rubber gloves if/when she had to do it herself).

We were told what Karen was to eat, with specific instructions from a dietician at the hospital. She was to eat lots of vegetables and grains. She was to drink bottled water—lots of it.

I was taught how to monitor Karen's blood sugar levels and to give her injections of insulin. Insulin was to be taken 30 minutes before eating and at a specific time at bedtime. It was expected the need for insulin would be for a fairly short time, however in some transplant patients, we were told, it has to be continued.

There was a hand-out called "Daily Schedule" with twelve items on it for us to follow; there was an alternate "Daily Schedule" hand-out with fifteen items on it for us to follow on "lab days" (that is, on days Karen would be going to the Mayo hospital to give blood after fasting, and also seeing various nurses and doctors.)

Karen was to be militant about her routine, including naps in the morning and naps in the afternoon. She was going to be on pain medication for the first four weeks. After that, she could use acetaminophen for pain. In no case was she to take aspirin, ibuprofen or any blood thinners (unless prescribed by the Mayo team).

She would not be able to eat grapefruit ever again and was told not to drink grapefruit juice or Fresca or anything with grapefruit juice in it (as it interferes with the effectiveness of some drugs).

Karen was told to ask the pharmacist each month for refills *before* her medications were completely used up.

She was told not to take any over-the-counter medicine, supplements, or herbs without checking with Jodie first.

During the teaching session, Jodie said it was her job to help Karen keep her new liver and to stay healthy. She also said it was her job to teach her to honor the donor family's decision to donate this organ. Jodie said there is a request that Mayo makes of each recipient. It is to write a letter to the donor family to thank them for their decision to donate. Jodie said it would be something she would talk with Karen about over the next weeks and months, and, when written, that the letter would be submitted to Jodie and forwarded, through channels, to the donor family.

All three of us took several moments to reflect on the donor family before we continued our discussion. Their loss of a loved one and their ultimate generosity changed Karen's life and the lives of others who received organs from just one person.

Chapter 18

Discharge from Hospital

I'm a list-maker and record-keeper, and I wanted to set up a system in the early days of Karen's post-transplant care that I could follow, and later share with Marcia to use as time went on.

On Friday, April 28, 2006 Karen was told there was *not* any cancer in the tumor that was in her own liver (that had been removed). That was great news, and we could put that worry to rest.

She was discharged from the hospital that day. Paul drove home to Alamogordo. After a quick trip to the grocery store, I prepared dinner for the two of us and got my patient settled into her new home-away-from-home at the Arizona Transplant House. We had moved into Room 3, which was the master bedroom of Brusally Ranch in its day. Ted and Donna (director and assistant director at the Transplant House, angels, both) provided a riser seat for the toilet and a walker for Karen's use, as her leg muscles were still weak. It was about then that I realized she should have had a riser seat on her toilets at home for at least six months *prior* to surgery.

Over and over I kept reminding myself not to feel overwhelmed. At that point all the many caregiver duties were squarely on my shoulders.

Jodie had given Karen a five-day supply of medications in a pillbox that had 28 compartments: four for each of the seven days of the week and further broken down for morning, noon, supper, bedtime (or perhaps breakfast, lunch, dinner, bedtime, some words like that.)

Karen had her first itinerary of blood work labs on Sunday, April 30. While we were at the Mayo Hospital we stopped at the pharmacy where she purchased a one-month supply of her medications.

Following her surgery Karen was still pretty weak. So we developed a routine: she would walk to the car with a walker and get into the front seat. I would then put the walker in the trunk and drive. Once at the Mayo Hospital entrance, I would park temporarily in the Unloading Only zone, then help Karen get seated in a wheelchair, leaving her in the airy, bright atrium. Then I would drive to a parking place, walk in from the parking lot, and finally push her to her scheduled appointments. We had to leave the Transplant House at least thirty to forty minutes before the earliest appointment, as each of those portions of the trip took time. I did a lot of walking. It always struck me as funny during that time when Karen would say, "It's time to run to my next appointment." She was never moving that fast!

On April 30th I lined up all the pill bottles. I carefully filled the pillbox for the next week, memorizing the color and shape of the various pills, checking and double-checking the dosages list. Jodie had instructed us that Marcia or I should fill the pillbox for a while, and that the weekly task of filling the pillbox would become Karen's responsibility after a few weeks.

Jodie had told us the immunosuppressive drugs were the most important, in fact, that they were as important to Karen's daily routine as clothing or glasses. She would be required to take them (or others that would be prescribed instead) for the rest of her life. Jodie had described the possible side effects for all the pills Karen would be taking. For example, some drugs cause other issues, like high blood pressure. So Karen had to take another medication for a while to keep her blood pressure low.

On Sunday, April 30th Karen woke from an afternoon nap. She said she was one of three people in a research lab and no one else was around. Then she said "they" were going on a trip and "she was in charge".

"And I remember thinking" she said, "what do I know about the Amazon?"

"I'm going to have to write this down!" I said. I remembered Jodie mentioning that a person could hallucinate from some of the drugs, so I asked Karen if she was hallucinating.

"It was a hallucination," she answered promptly.

"In that case," I replied, "I'm going to have to call Jodie."

"Oh, it was probably just a dream; I'd better not close my eyes" Karen said. Minutes later, she was asleep again. I knew she was on some really powerful drugs, so I watched her carefully for the rest of the afternoon.

On Tuesday, May 2, 2006 Karen and I got up, dressed, and out early for her next labs and scheduled appointments at Mayo. I took a notebook with me, and I'm glad I did. I honestly do not know how a patient (who is less than 2 weeks past her [or his] date of surgery) or a caregiver can *possibly* remember all the information any other way.

Jodie gave Karen some instructions on how her insurance would pay for some of the expensive prescription drugs. Based on the results of the blood work, her dosage for Prograf was reduced. Prograf is one of the immunosuppressive drugs she was taking. An additional antiviral medication was added, and we were told the prescription for it was waiting in the pharmacy. Karen was directed to wear compression socks, at least for 3 weeks, because of the swelling in her legs.

Dr. Brown met with Karen and me next. He said her platelet count was better, that 200 was a normal reading, but hers was 293. He told her to follow a low sodium diet, due to the swelling in her legs and feet. He commented on the fact that Karen received a "split liver" and that the other portion, approximately 25%, went to a baby in California. He said her liver numbers following transplant (during which the organ gets shocked) were coming down nicely. He warned of possible complications, such as an infection, a blood clot (in Karen's case because of the Greenfield filter), a problem with bile ducts, or abnormal kidney function, and explained those were the primary reasons why she had to be seen twice a week. I forced myself not to worry about those things; we would face them only if or when something happened.

He told Karen to drink a *gallon* of water every day. He said he would be prescribing Coumadin, but would call with the appropriate dose. He said Karen lost seventeen units of blood during the surgery, which I thought was a lot. But the discussion continued, and I kept listing the items mentioned. Karen's wound was healing well, she was told, and the staples were to come out in about 2 weeks. It was a lot of information. But to my ears and thinking, it sounded like everything was looking pretty good on the tenth day after surgery.

That afternoon Lea's friend Marcia arrived from Mississippi. She had arranged to get a ride from the airport, which was a big deal to me; I was thrilled that I didn't have to drive to Phoenix to pick her up. Marcia was a tremendous "breath of fresh air" in so many ways. Her Southern accent was a delight to our ears. She was enthusiastic about being in the desert southwest and about her ability to care for Karen. She had actually met Karen years before. She viewed her as someone who had just had a major surgery and was on the mend. She knew of Karen through Lea's eyes, and thought of her as an accomplished, talented woman, which she is. Sadly, that view was not what I'd been concentrating on during recent weeks while she had been getting increasingly sicker, so it was important for me to view Karen through Marcia's eyes and to begin to switch my thinking to a more optimistic view for Karen's recovery.

For obvious reasons, Marcia didn't have my memories of how ill Karen had been in February and March. She observed that Karen was using a walker, but was able to get around on her own. Marcia's personality is positive, and she focused on what Karen could do, and encouraged her to do more. Marcia is a good cook, and volunteered to take over that duty immediately, which was an enormous relief to me, as anything to do with cooking is not my strong suit.

For the next eleven days, Marcia and I cared for Karen together. Having both of us there was a blessing for everyone.

On Thursday, May 4th Karen arose early and walked to the opposite end of the house to the room where a scale was located. Her weight was 173.2 pounds, still very high for a woman who is 5'3" tall. Some of the post-transplant drugs she was taking caused swelling and edema. I remember thinking to myself that Karen's body had learned how to retain fluids extremely well during the previous years. Even though we had met other liver transplant patients who appeared to be fit and slim, it seemed it was going to take time for Karen's body to change.

After the routine labs Karen, Marcia and I followed her appointment schedule to a meeting with Dr. Brown. I made another list; this time there were twenty items on it. Much of it was a repeat of Karen's twice-a-week routine, such as reminders to pick up a new itinerary each time we were at Mayo. We also heard the doctor's reactions and comments about Karen's statistics from The Three-Ring-Binder [a proper noun because we all used and consulted The Binder so many times through Karen's convalescence. The information contained in it provided many of the details for this section of this book].

Karen reported itching and the doctor said there were several reasons why it could be happening. He said the prescription drug for pain sometimes caused itching, but since she had been taking it for two weeks by then, he didn't think she was allergic to it. He said her bilyrubin[21] level was normal and that her new liver was producing bile the way a liver is supposed to produce it. He suggested that we wash the bed sheets again, using mild laundry soap. He advised Karen to use a mild bar soap in the shower, and to use lukewarm water, not hot water. He said she could begin to take some antihistamine the following week if the itching was still bothering her then.

Karen was told her temperature and blood pressure readings looked good. The doctor noted she did not have "auto-immune hepatitis" so she would *not* have to continue taking Prednisone indefinitely. He reminded Marcia and me that the Prednisone taper schedule <u>would not</u> change and that we should follow the diminishing dosages precisely until the schedule ended. He said we could pick up a new medication diary (unique to Karen, based on new prescriptions each visit) from the front desk.

When we asked about Physical Therapy, since Karen was not very active or strong yet, we were told insurance would not cover it. So it became another task for her caregivers. I obtained an exercise handout we could follow. The next day I began conducting exercise sessions with Karen at the dining room table at the Transplant House.

Dr. Brown told Karen to make an appointment with her local gastroenterologist when she got home to Green Valley and to make friends with him or her. He instructed her to explain about her liver transplant, that Mayo would be directing her care, and that Mayo would continue to coordinate with the gastroenterologist from then on into the future.

Karen was told to get a pneumonia shot after 4 months. She was reminded that her sodium intake should be 2,000 mg per day or less. Karen had been following a low sodium diet for years, so this was not a problem. She was told her kidney function was sub optimal (or subnormal or a word like that) and that her creatinine level was slightly elevated. Dr. Brown said the creatinine level would need to come down and that Karen was not drinking enough water. He said she should drink a gallon of water a day and suggested using a straw to drink more.

Dr. Brown noted the swelling in Karen's legs was worse, that she had more fluid in her abdomen, and said it was likely there was also fluid in her lungs, called pleural effusions. Because of all this, he said he was going to add a diuretic to Karen's list of medications. He told Karen to take one a day to begin, and he would review her fluid situation again the following week. He said she would be okay taking a diuretic because her potassium level was "high normal" and she could afford to let it decrease a little (as the diuretic would deplete her potassium level). He also suggested that Karen should do some deep breathing exercises a couple of times each day.

As noted two days earlier, Karen's so-called liver numbers were coming down, as they were supposed to do after transplant surgery. Of the various numbers they looked at, two were normal and the others were trending down, which also sounded good. An ultrasound had been performed 5 days after transplant; another one was scheduled for the next day, May 5th. The platelet count (which was slightly elevated two days earlier) was higher still (now 420), and the doctor said he wasn't sure why it had gone up even more. He said it might have had something to do with the anti-rejection drug, and it was possible Karen was not tolerating her current dosage well. He said he would change the mix of drugs, and would call Karen with the new dosages.

Dr. Brown described the reasons to call Jodie or to go to the Emergency Room: fever, shaking chills, drenching sweats (all signs of infection), nausea, vomiting, diarrhea, abnormal bleeding, very uncomfortable swelling, bad headache, or generally feeling unwell. He said, "Do not wait." It was a good review for Karen and me, and it was good for Marcia to hear these instructions for the first time.

The doctor said it was time for Karen to increase her activity level more. He said her activities should include going to the bathroom, showering, walking, making her own meals, reading, sitting up with her feet elevated, etc., instead of spending so much time in bed. Perhaps we were trying to be protective of Karen, but neither Marcia nor I mentioned at that point how little Karen was doing in terms of activity two weeks after her transplant surgery.

That was a mistake.

Karen responded best to orders from a doctor or someone in a position of authority, and I don't think enough emphasis was given to how much she *should have been doing* at that juncture in her recovery.

The doctor said he would be prescribing Coumadin, which would shift the balance in Karen's blood and prevent clotting around her filter. He said he would start her on a low dose and monitor it closely. The doctor said Karen should be off all her prescription pain medication (she was on Percocet) by week 6. He said her pain would likely increase the next two to three weeks, but that she should try to get by with as little pain medicine as possible. He said to take no more than four doses of Percocet per day. I had noticed it seemed to make Karen even more sluggish, so I asked if using Tylenol during the day and Percocet at night would be okay. Dr. Brown said, yes, that would be fine, so I made a note in The Binder to change the routine immediately. Incidentally, Karen never complained much about pain.

Over the weekend Marcia and I left Karen alone in her room at the Transplant House for a little more than an hour while we went to a grocery store. When we got back Karen said, "You abandoned me!" At first I felt bad; then I thought it might be a good sign that my very social sister-in-law felt like she was missing out on something we were doing. I was both amazed and disappointed to hear her say that she had stayed in her chair the entire time we were gone, not even getting up to use the bathroom or stroll around the room.

Karen knew she was supposed to be getting regular exercise but still wasn't doing it on her own. Much later I learned Karen was frustrated because she wanted to be active and to improve, but she simply didn't have the strength and stamina. It didn't help to see others at the Transplant House improving steadily while she seemed to be on a plateau with little or no improvement from day to day.

During the next week Karen had her regular Tuesday session starting with blood work in the early morning, followed by doctor visits throughout the day. One of the people Karen visited with was a psychologist. He asked Karen how she felt she was doing. In response Karen related that she was tremendously frustrated with her progress, that she wished she could be walking more and doing more, but that she just didn't seem to have much energy. The doctor asked if she was sad, angry, or frustrated.

"I need to tell my brother Paul to back off!" she said forcefully. This vehement statement seemed to come out of the blue! Marcia and I exchanged a quick look of surprise. For some reason Karen had decided to place all her frustration on her brother. Gone were the days when Karen wanted to please Paul with her progress. That day she had trouble articulating how motivated *she wanted to be*, that in her recovery phase she just didn't have the energy.

Unfortunately her discussion about how Paul had been trying to encourage her on the phone took the focus off how little she was actually moving around. Neither Karen, Marcia, nor I knew how to ask, "Is this normal?" or, "Is there something else going on that is affecting how I'm doing?" I know she wanted to bounce back more quickly than she was doing, and I wanted that, too.

"He's not here, and he doesn't understand," she added, talking about Paul's coaching again.

The doctor soothed Karen, suggesting she seemed to be a perfectionist and that it was okay to cut herself some slack. Karen said she never wanted to be an invalid again. The doctor reminded her that she had always been motivated to follow instructions and to get well.

"And I am trying," she emphasized. That was all she was able to say right then.

When he understood that Karen's brother was also my husband, the doctor made a point of suggesting to me that Paul should be told not to push so hard. I obediently assured him, "I will talk to Paul." The doctor told Karen not to overreact to the fact that she was not having a perfect course toward recovery and that it was still less than three weeks since her transplant. That seemed to calm Karen down, giving her permission, in a way, to be slow and cautious about her activity level, if that suited her.

We were all impatient to see Karen's condition improve dramatically, but it wasn't happening that way. I was remembering the man from Pinetop who had gone home three weeks after his surgery. It saddened me at that point that Karen did not seem to understand what a huge role Paul had played in the previous many weeks, working with doctors and nurses, moving her from Tucson to Phoenix, and helping to keep her reasonably well so she could be reactivated and eligible for her transplant surgery. I also knew Paul is tough, and he could take it if Karen was going to make him the scapegoat for her frustration right then. For the time being, we had to be content with the doctor appointments where we heard Karen's liver numbers and some other issues *were* trending nicely.

That day we also met with Jodie, who reviewed Karen's weight (180.6) and blood pressure (128/84). Jodie said the slightly elevated blood pressure and fluid build-up was fairly typical, especially since Karen had experienced a lot of fluid build-up before transplant as well.

"You have no ankles," Jodie exclaimed. She said Karen should continue taking the diuretic. Karen's immunosuppressive drug dose was to be lowered. The elevated level of that drug (as indicated by that day's lab tests) could have been because Karen was dehydrated, because of low blood sugar, or because of her elevated blood pressure.

In terms of exercise, Jodie said Karen should do "what you can" and that she "should do it more often". Jodie said, "You will only get better as you develop more stamina and strength."

When we visited with Dr. Clarke, she said Karen would not be released to go home to Green Valley until she could walk on her own without a walker. She urged Karen to stop thinking about herself as a sick person and to concentrate on being well. I thought this was *huge*. Karen had viewed herself as sick for years and it would take a big paradigm shift for her to think otherwise.

Both Jodie and Dr. Clarke said Karen's kidney function had gotten worse and instructed her to drink more fluids. Those instructions did seem confusing at a time when the fluid build-up in her abdomen and ankles was high. Both Marcia and I routinely battled with Karen to drink more. We all were told we had to be patient, to let the various medications work. We were reminded that with more time we *would* see the extra fluid come off.

Chapter 19

Emergency Room Visit

On Thursday, May 11ᵗʰ Marcia got up early to walk with Karen to the other end of the house for her morning weigh-in. Karen seemed to be out of breath before she even made it across the room. By the time they returned, she was gasping for air and said she simply couldn't get her breath. Fortunately, Ted Dailey was in the office of the Transplant House early that day, and provided a wheelchair. As Marcia helped Karen put on her shoes, I phoned Jodie at Mayo to report Karen's symptoms. Since I was unable to reach Jodie for further instruction, Marcia, Ted and I had a quick consultation and decided it was appropriate to take Karen to the Mayo Emergency Room.

Several hours later we were back in our room at the Transplant House. Karen's fluid build-up, this time in her chest cavity, was indeed pressing on her lungs and making it difficult to breathe. The ER staff performed a procedure called a thoracentesis, removing fluid from the area around Karen's lungs. She said later the procedure was painful. She also said once the fluid was gone there was immediate relief.

Marcia was quite upset by this crisis. She had envisioned a crisis-free, steady improvement after surgery. I was able to calm her down with some of the same words I had shared with Karen in the past. We were so lucky to be close to the ER, to be "in the Mayo system" and to have access to knowledgeable people who had treated other transplant patients before and knew just what to do. I didn't want to sound like I wasn't concerned because I absolutely was. But it was definitely not the first crisis I'd been through with Karen. I was confident she had just received proper care and would be followed closely over the next few days. In fact, that afternoon we received a call from Jodie and were told to increase Karen's dosage of her diuretic; clearly she needed more medication and the excess fluid in her body needed to come off.

Back in our room Karen said she was exhausted. Off and on throughout the afternoon Marcia and I urged her to get up and walk around the room a little, but she wasn't moving. She acted like she didn't remember or didn't need to heed Jodie's advice about exercising at least a little bit but quite often, which she had heard the day before. Maybe she had decided to concentrate on Jodie's other instructions, "Do what you can" and felt she couldn't do anything. Both Marcia and I had heard Karen say, "I can't" many times over the previous week and a half. Later that day Karen had to walk to the dining room for her supper (it was a house rule not to serve any meals in the rooms), so she got a tiny amount of exercise then.

I was frustrated for a couple of reasons. It was not easy for me to be patient about Karen's lack of exercise. When she had been at the nursing home, she would go to physical therapy and do the things she was asked by a stranger. Now that it was Marcia or me urging her to get moving she did not respond. In addition, I was scheduled to go home on Saturday. I was torn. Marcia was on board and doing a great job. But I really wanted to see Karen "turn a corner" and really improve before I went home.

Fortunately, Karen was a little more energetic on Friday. Marcia had suggested a trip to a nearby drugstore, and once again, "shopping therapy" worked very well. That day, using a shopping cart for balance, Karen strolled around the store for around 30 minutes, and purchased some more cosmetics. On Saturday morning Karen and Marcia had fun applying makeup and fussing with their hair while I packed my bags. All their relaxed activity, which seemed so normal, simply the two of them enjoying each other's company, helped me get in touch with the thought that it was okay for me to go. Marcia really was good for Karen, and I finally began to know that the women in Room 3 at the Transplant House were going to be fine.

Paul drove to Scottsdale on May 13th, arriving around 4 p.m. Karen wore a yellow over-shirt that day, and looked good, although she was still very heavy. The two of them had a private conversation for about ten minutes on the patio before I even knew Paul was there. Paul stayed for about an hour, meeting Marcia, grabbing a quick nap, and having another talk with Karen.

I couldn't sit still. I still had some packing to finish, and wandered around the house, saying goodbye to the other guests. When Paul said it was time to go, Karen and I had a tearful goodbye. It had been six months since the day after Thanksgiving when I drove Karen home in her car. We had been through so much since then.

Karen, Paul and I kept in touch by telephone. Marcia and I kept in touch for a while with text-messages and by phone. I think that Marcia hated to see me go; it was easier to care for Karen when there were two of us to share the many (often stressful) tasks. Karen continued to have appointments at Mayo twice a week. She did not join in with cooking or doing her own laundry, and Marcia said she was very slow at showering or getting dressed each day. Marcia continued driving Karen to her appointments, caring for her, recording and supervising medication doses, cooking, doing laundry and all the other chores that needed to be done, all the while trying not to feel overwhelmed. She often mentioned that she had to concentrate on one day at a time.

At the end of May Karen insisted to her doctors that something "just wasn't right". She described her various symptoms, and a thyroid test was ordered. This was an important turning point. It had been too easy to blame Karen for being lethargic and not working harder at walking and becoming stronger. Karen knew something was wrong, her doctors listened, and called for another blood test. Also, some of my research revealed the following: "About one in ten people with chronic hepatitis C have antibodies to their own thyroid gland, which can lead to a sluggish thyroid (hypothyroidism)."[22]

Karen was one of those patients, and was immediately given a prescription for synthetic thyroid hormone. Within just a few days, she reported her energy returned, she didn't feel as cold all the time, and she began walking greater distances. With her increase of activity, the fluid built up in tissues throughout her body started to diminish, and she began to lose weight. Finally a significant improvement everyone was waiting for in Karen's recovery came about.

As promised, Dr. Clarke, Dr. Brown and Jodie Gonzalez didn't release Karen to go home to Green Valley until she was ready. Some of the members of her family were scheduled to come for a visit, so their arrival became an additional motivation for her to be able to show them how well she was doing.

Lea was coming with her niece Caroline and nephew Ron, (Karen's grandchildren). They arrived in Phoenix on June 17th. They were able to stay in the Phoenix area for two nights and visit Karen at the Arizona Transplant House. Then on June 20th Marcia, Lea, and the kids took her home.

As scheduled, Marcia went home to Mississippi on June 27, 2006. She had fulfilled her eight-week commitment and nursed Karen through a long and significant portion of her recovery.

Karen's friend Grace flew in and stayed with Karen for another month after that. Both women realized after a very short amount of time that Karen was ready to be on her own. However, Grace stayed as promised for four weeks. Karen was on her own by the end of July 2006.

Karen's son Randy visited his mom in August.

Karen had come through an amazing period in her life. And she continues to prosper. At the time this book was ready to be published and five years after the transplant, she was doing extremely well. Occasionally she has been instructed to decrease her immunosuppressive drugs somewhat again. She's walking and exercising to stay fit.

If someone meets her for the first time, they have no idea Karen has ever been ill. She is energetic and living life to the fullest. She has joined various social organizations and continues to be active in her church.

"I'm so busy!" is her frequent remark.

She doesn't waste a day. She fills her time with activities that delight her. She is a good mother, sister, sister-in-law, and friend to many people all over the country. She knows she has been given a remarkable gift and does not squander it.

Chapter 20

Reflections

Donor Family: It took the selfless gift of a donor family in the time of their incomprehensible grief to make a liver available for Karen (as well as other organs for recipients who benefited from this family's tragic loss). I believe Karen was one of 6 recipients who gained a new organ (or a portion of an organ).

Medical Community: It took the dedicated and professional team at Mayo, who performs miracles every day. Before Dr. Clarke's pep talk in the Mayo Hospital March 18th (a full month before her transplant) Karen did not seem to understand the importance of becoming mobile again or that *she* had the power to get stronger. That was a significant turning point. In addition, it took Dr. Cho and the physical therapy staff at the Scottsdale nursing home, as well as the staff at the Tucson rehab center before that, and countless nameless medical people at the Tucson ER who treated Karen and got her through various medical events and crises. It had all begun with Karen's doctor in Mississippi, who aided Karen in extending her liver function through medication and diet when Karen was first diagnosed (and for years until she moved to Arizona).

Caregivers: It took a team of people to help Karen through her ordeal, starting with the devotion of Dave and her children when Karen was diagnosed with Hepatitis C in 1999. It took the companionship of Dave's cousin Norma when Karen first started to go to Mayo in Phoenix for her transplant evaluation appointments. It took Penny's unhesitating willingness to stay with Karen for nearly three months (just eight months after her own back surgery). It took Paul and me stepping in when it seemed there was no one else to guide the process. It took my ability to move to Scottsdale, and our concentration on Karen's needs to convince everyone at the Transplant House and on the Mayo team that we were indeed her committed caregivers. It took Lea's focus on finding her mother another caregiver and Marcia's cheerful personality to take over Karen's care after Paul and I moved on. It took the friendship of Grace to come to Green Valley and be sure Karen was well enough to be on her own.

The Patient: It took Karen's unwavering focus on becoming one of the lucky few who does indeed get a transplant, as well as her extraordinary will to live to get her through her amazing and difficult medical ordeal. Karen had entered the first rehab center on January 30, 2006. Against extremely long odds, on April 21, 2006 she received her liver transplant. A little more than two months later, she was at home. By July Karen's weight was down from an all-time high of 205 pounds to 126 pounds. She was slim and well.

My January dream about her walking toward me, smiling, and healthy had finally come true.

Epilogue

There were so many things that we learned along the way. Here are some of the musings I've had since our family's experience:

If not for the generosity of the family of the donor, Karen would not be alive. Karen wrote her letter of gratitude about a year after surgery, and it was forwarded to the mother of the teenager who had died in April 2006. Karen and I met the young woman's mother in April 2008. Because of our respect for their family's privacy, I have decided not to write much about them, other than to say they know the depth of Karen's gratitude and the thanks from the rest of the family, especially Paul and me, who saw her go to the very brink of not making it.

There were dozens of people who helped Karen along the way. Many of us knew Karen and could not imagine life without her. Others, in the various medical and rehabilitation facilities, only came to know her through her illness and recovery. She needed each and every one of them at the time they came into her life, and it is miraculous to realize how all of them and their assistance contributed to the reality of Karen's new lease on life. There were many specific events for Karen that, if they had not happened the way they did, she would not have made it.

We all wish Karen could have avoided becoming so ill. It is a cruel irony that a patient has to be nearer to death than other candidates in order to be the one chosen for a transplant. If we could have known that she was going to feel bad, and weak, but that she should have been walking around the house and around her neighborhood *anyway*, perhaps her last few months before transplant would not have been so difficult. Staying active was critical.

As a disease progresses, the patient and her family members often are more knowledgeable about liver failure (or some other life-threatening disease) than the people they meet in doctors' offices and emergency rooms. Every patient and caregiver involved must not hesitate to inform and instruct people as needed about the peculiar needs of the patient. Be assertive and persistent. Hone your management skills. Manage the medical community for the best outcome for the patient. Be prepared to state things more than once in case someone doesn't want to listen or doesn't want to learn from you.

Some families have to move (temporarily or permanently) to another city or another state to be near their transplant facility or specialized medical center. Choose a location that is within one hour or less of that location as your base.

Do your homework. Some hospitals are better than others. Mayo is outstanding.

As the patient, as soon as possible and every day, develop your will to live. Fill the universe with your positive thoughts and the outcome you desire; the universe will deliver. Focus on the positive outcome, which for Karen was a successful transplant and good health. Karen never said, "If I get a new liver", she always said "When I get a new liver." She had an unwavering conviction that she would be selected and that she would get well. She had developed that conviction in 1986 when she defeated an advanced kind of cancer; she renewed that conviction in 2006 when she needed a liver transplant.

As caregivers, challenge the patients. Challenge them to remain active. Challenge their minds. Encourage them to think of themselves as normal people with serious illnesses. Encourage them to live as "normally" as possible. Become involved with medications early in the process and don't let the routine vary. Follow dietary recommendations and don't cheat. I walked on eggshells around Karen, not wanting to upset her. Paul made her stretch. He convinced her that finding additional caregivers was her challenge and encouraged her to make phone calls and explore options. It was good for her to use her mind and to be involved in that process.

As caregivers, know when to ask for help. Take a break. Go to the library. Get a haircut. It's okay to feel overwhelmed; when you do, write a list, take a walk, and, if it is in your belief system, pray. Ask someone else to come in and sit with the patient, if that is needed, and be specific about what you need. "I need to go out for 2 hours on Tuesday at 10 a.m." is much clearer than, "Why don't you come over sometime so I can get out of the house for a while?" People will be happy to help when they know exactly what you need.

It may also be interesting to note that you're reinvigorated and ready to get back to the patient. After my shopping day away from Karen at IKEA, it was fascinating for me to realize that even though I had been exhausted, both mentally and physically most of the time, I was also anxious to get back to her.

Watch the interaction between the patient and some of the people that visit. If someone seems to make the patient "perk up" (as Paul always did with Karen), be sure you get that person to visit often.

As a patient, say Thank You. Say it like you mean it. It goes a long way toward keeping everyone's spirits up. Know that you may need several devoted caregivers, not just one. Being sick is tough. Being a caregiver can be tougher.

From the beginning I was fascinated by Karen's story. How awful to have defeated cancer, and wind up with Hepatitis and liver failure. I always wanted the best outcome for her. But becoming involved with the crisis that was her failing health and unknown future was one of the most frustrating and scary periods of my life. To be able to step in, by default and reluctantly, was an amazing and life-changing experience for all of us.

I have often thought about the book I might have written, changing history to show Karen as a willing and serene patient even through those awful days of hepatic encephalopathy, Paul as a devoted brother and myself as a selfless sister-in-law. But families don't always work the way they might in a scripted Hollywood feel-good movie. In the final analysis, Karen was determined, and Grace, Marcia, Penny, Paul and I were extremely capable. We all did the best we could, and we were so lucky. For our entire family, Karen's successful transplant and continuing good health is our reward and our triumph.

Call For Action:

Finally, look into becoming a donor. The need is far greater than the number of organs that are available.[23]

Endnotes

1   www.medicinenet.com/hodgkins_disease.htm

2   Turkington, Carol. *Hepatitis C The Silent Killer*, Contemporary Books, 1998, p. 9.

3   Author's Note: Another person with a Hepatitis C diagnosis should follow his or her doctor's orders.

4   http://health.yahoo.com/hepatitis-treatment/hepatitis-c-treatment-overview//healthwise—aa132906.html

5   Turkington, op. cit. p. xvii.

6   Ibid. p. 20.

7   Ibid. p. xi.

8   Ibid. pp. 4, 12.

9   Turkington, p. 4.

10   Ibid. p. 12.

11   Ibid. p. 16.

12   "Interferon is a protein that is naturally produced in your body to fight infection; alpha interferon is an artificially produced copy of the natural protein." "The drug both interferes with virus reproduction and stimulates the immune system to fight infections." Turkington, p. 58.

13   www.optn.transplant.hrsa.gov Organ Procurement and Transplantation Network. When I visited the website on December 22, 2010, it showed the following: waiting list candidates 110,345. Active waiting list candidates, 72,670. Transplants done between January and September 2010, 21,648. Donors during January and September 2010, 10,940.
www.unos.org Visited website on various dates.

14   www.webmed.com/heartburn-gerd/guide/upper-endoscopy Visited website on various dates.

15 Turkington, pp. 86-87.

16 http://en.wikipedia.org/wiki/Hepatitis_C Visited website on various dates.

17 www.unos.org website. "The United Network for Organ Sharing (UNOS), a non-profit charitable organization, operates the Organ Procurement and Transplantation Network (OPTN) under federal contract. On an ongoing basis, the OPTN/UNOS evaluates new advances and research and adapts these into new policies to best serve patients waiting for transplants."

"As part of this process, the OPTN/UNOS developed a system for prioritizing candidates waiting for liver transplants based on statistical formulas that are very accurate for predicting who needs a liver transplant most urgently. The MELD (Model for End Stage Liver Disease) is used for candidates age 12 and older and the PELD (Pediatric End Stage Liver Disease Model) is used for patients age 11 and younger."

"This document will explain the system and how it affects those needing a transplant."

"What is MELD? How is it used?" "The Model for End-Stage Liver Disease (MELD) is a numerical scale, ranging from 6 (less ill) to 40 (gravely ill), used for liver transplant candidates age 12 and older. It gives each person a 'score' (number) based on how urgently he or she needs a liver transplant within the next three months. The number is calculated by a formula using three routine lab test results: Bilyrubin, which measures how effectively the liver excretes bile; INR (prothrombin time), which measures the liver's ability to make blood clotting factors; and creatinine, which measures kidney function. (Impaired kidney function is often associated with severe liver disease.)"

"The only priority exception to MELD is a category known as Status 1. Status 1 patients have acute (sudden and severe) onset liver failure and a life expectancy of hours to a few days without transplant. All other liver candidates age 12 and older are prioritized by the MELD system."

"A patient's score may go up or down over time depending on the status of his or her liver disease. Most candidates will have their MELD score assessed a number of times while they are on a waiting list. This will help ensure that donated livers go to the patients in greatest need at that moment."

18 Author's Note: I do not believe Karen would have lived through another six months. There were many clues to this reality Paul and I did not concentrate on at the time. We were so focused on getting through the day or getting some resolution to the current crisis that we didn't stop to add them all up. Among them were her diminished condition during and after the trip to Europe, her talkative, social personality change, her two trips to the Emergency Room in January, the blood clot business, Jack's plea for her children to come for a visit, and Karen's exhaustion and increasingly frequent daytime naps.

19 www.Healthwise.com "Albumin is a protein that is made in the liver and released into the blood. It helps prevent blood from leaking out of blood vessels, and it carries medications and other substances through the blood. When albumin levels drop, fluid may collect in the ankles (pedal edema), lungs (pulmonary edema), or belly (ascites)."

20 Author's Note: Discharge instructions were written at the time of Jodie's teaching session and I am not in the medical profession so they could be wrong. Another patient should not follow the instructions included here. They are included only to illustrate that post-operative care for a transplant patient is complicated.

21 Turkington, p. 32. "Bilyrubin is an orange to yellow pigment in bile that is the result of the breakdown of hemoglobin. Too much bilyrubin produces jaundice and is a sign of liver damage."

22 Turkington, p. 96.

23 www.transplantfundation.org Myths Busted: Myth: Doctors may let a patient die so they can transplant organs to their other patients. Fact: Doctors who treat patients at the time of death have nothing to do with donation or transplantation of those organs and tissues. Every effort is made to save the patient's life before donation can be considered.

Myth: Donating organs and tissues goes against religious beliefs. Fact: All major religions support donation and have provided statements for their members. [The website has a link for a listing of religions and their affiliation to organ donation.]

Myth: Transplants don't really work. They're experimental. Fact: Transplantation is a standard medical procedure, and one year survival rates for kidney recipients are almost 96%; for heart recipients, over 86%, for liver recipients 86%.

Myth: Donation is painful for the donor's family. Fact: Studies show that donation most often provides immediate and long-term consolation. Donation can be especially comforting when the death is unexpected and the donor is young.

Myth: It costs money to donate. Fact: Donor families are not charged for the medical costs associated with organ and tissue donation.

Myth: Wealthy people can buy organs. Fact: It's a federal crime to buy or sell organs. For people on the national waiting list for organs, matching is based on blood and tissue type, medical urgency, time on the waiting list, and geographical location. There is no way to buy a place on the national waiting list.

Myth: Donation disfigures the body and delays the funeral. Fact: Donation surgery includes careful reconstruction of the body and doesn't interfere with funeral plans, including open-casket services. Most donations take place within 24 hours after death, so funeral arrangements will not be delayed.

Myth: Signing a donor card is pointless. Fact: Signing a donor card, and discussing your decision with family members, is the best way to assure that your personal wishes will be carried out.

Transplant Foundation, Inc., 701 SW 27th Avenue, Suite 705, Miami, FL 33135.